Overcoming Common Problems

The PMS Handbook

Natural ways to balance your hormones

Theresa Cheung

D1585961

sheldon **PRESS**

First published in Great Britain in 2006

Sheldon Press
36 Causton Street
London SW1P 4ST

The author and publisher have made every effort to ensure
that the external website and email addresses included in this book are
correct and up to date at the time of going to press. The author
and publisher are not responsible for the content, quality or
continuing accessibility of the sites.

British Library Cataloguing-in-Publication Data

A catalogue record for this book is available from the British Library

ISBN-13: 978–0–85969–984–8
ISBN-10: 0–85969–984–6

1 3 5 7 9 10 8 6 4 2

Typeset by Deltatype Limited, Birkenhead, Merseyside
Printed in Great Britain by Ashford Colour Press

Contents

THE PM

THERESA CHEUNG i
popular psychology bool
All Evil, *Get Lucky: Mal*
Lazy Person's Guide to Stress and *Living with the
Glycaemic Factor* (Sheldon Press). She also co-authored
the best-selling *PCOS Diet Book* and has contributed
features to *Here's Health*, *NHS Mother and Baby*, *You Are
What You Eat*, *Red*, *She* and *Prima* magazines.

Overcoming Common Problems Series

Selected titles

A full list of titles is available from Sheldon Press,
36 Causton Street, London SW1P 4ST and on our website at
www.sheldonpress.co.uk

Introduction
Taking charge of the monthly roller-coaster

Headaches, bloating, a craving for sweets, irritability, crying and cramps are the all too familiar symptoms of PMS, or premenstrual syndrome, which is thought to affect a staggering 85 per cent of women in their childbearing years. Some 10 per cent of these women also experience conditions such as shakiness, self-harm and even suicidal thoughts.

There is plenty of information about PMS, but what women really want, to answer Freud, is to know how to control the condition. Doctors still disagree about the causes and treatment of PMS, and the latest thinking is that this is a much more individual condition than was previously believed – and far more multi-factorial, often necessitating a combination of approaches.

In spite of today's medical advances, scientists have still not found one cure for PMS. No single treatment exists for PMS, and what works for one woman may not work for another. There are, however, a number of proven ways to take charge of your health, balance your hormones and ease your symptoms and you'll find them all here. This practical book presents ten different approaches to PMS and, depending on your symptoms and their severity, you can benefit from using these singly or in combination. The topics covered include diet, supplements, exercise, natural progesterone, herbs, xenoestrogens, stress, light therapy, alternative therapies, and positive thinking. There's also a handy A to Z of the most common symptoms and natural ways to beat them. A good idea may be to experiment with all the suggestions offered in this book and find out what works best for you.

While medical help is covered in the chapters that follow, the emphasis is on finding natural ways to balance your hormones and offering suggestions as to what you yourself can do to stop the monthly roller-coaster. Whether you suffer from minor bloating, cramps and headaches, or major crying breakdowns, *The PMS Handbook* will help you conquer this often debilitating condition and make you feel wonderful every day of the month.

1

All about PMS

Do you keep crying for no reason at all? Are you happy one moment, but angry the next? Do you feel bloated, headachy and tired? Do you get such powerful cravings for chocolate or sweets that you simply cannot concentrate on anything else?

If you suffer from a variety of physical and emotional symptoms around the time of your period, then you may be among the millions of women worldwide who suffer from PMS. Though it is often joked about, PMS is no laughing matter. It can leave you feeling depressed, tired out, and unable to face the world.

It wasn't so long ago that many doctors and women's health experts insisted that PMS didn't really exist. It was all in your mind, they said. As a result, many women who suffered from this condition were led to believe that they were oversensitive, lazy, self-indulgent or just plain crazy. Thankfully, this isn't the case today and PMS is now recognized as a true health condition.

PMS certainly isn't all in your mind. It's painful, unpleasant and distressing. It can make you feel terrible. That's why you need to take it seriously and find ways to deal with it. How can you feel good about yourself and your life if you feel miserable, bloated and uncomfortable half the time?

The chapters that follow will show you ways to balance your hormones naturally and beat PMS, so it doesn't destroy the quality of much of your life. But before exploring self-help options, it is important to understand what PMS is and whether you actually have it or could be mistaking it for another condition.

What is PMS?

Premenstrual syndrome, or PMS, is a disorder characterized by a set of hormonal changes that can trigger a mixture of symptoms. These symptoms can affect your physical and emotional health and well-being for up to two weeks before your period. Typically, PMS tends to start about midway through your cycle (around day 14 or about the time of ovulation) and continues until your period has begun.

1

PMS can affect any woman at any time during her reproductive life and can interfere with normal activities at home, school or work. Recent research[1] has also indicated that during the premenstrual phase, activity in brain regions that help control emotions increases and may explain the feelings of vulnerability that many women experience at this time.

In short, PMS can wreak havoc on just about every area of your life: relationships, education, career, family, sex and friends. Menopause, when monthly periods stop, often brings an end to PMS.

What are the symptoms?

More than 150 PMS symptoms have been documented through various studies. Most women exhibit just a handful of these symptoms during their PMS; however, some women experience up to a dozen or more at one time. The most common symptoms are listed below and they include bloating, breast tenderness, constipation, fatigue, food cravings, clumsiness and mood swings. You may or may not have the same set of symptoms each month and some months may be worse than others. Your symptoms may also be very different from someone else's. The variations are endless.

How PMS can affect your body:
- Breast swelling and tenderness
- Abdominal bloating
- Swollen ankles, feet or hands
- Fluid retention
- Back pain
- Headache
- Migraines
- Trouble sleeping
- Abdominal cramps
- Low energy/fatigue
- Acne breakouts
- Cold sores
- Constipation/diarrhoea or nausea
- Appetite changes and food cravings
- Joint or muscle pain/stiffness
- Dizziness

2

- Sweating
- Rapid heartbeat

How PMS can affect your emotions:
- Moodiness
- Irritability
- Crying spells
- Feeling anxious
- Sadness
- Feeling tense
- Lack of interest in daily activities
- Forgetfulness
- Confusion
- Difficulty in concentrating
- Anger/aggression
- Panic attacks
- Fearfulness/paranoia
- Difficulty handling stress
- Feeling out of control
- Decreased self-esteem
- Change in sexual desire
- Withdrawal from others

PMDD and PMM

For most women, PMS is irritating and unpleasant, but for others it can be a severely debilitating disorder. In fact, in a tiny percentage of cases – between 2 and 9 per cent – symptoms are so severe they become destructive, and women have to rearrange their work, school or social schedules around their PMS. This severe form of PMS is called PMDD – premenstrual dysphoric disorder. PMDD generally lasts longer than PMS, and for some women it can wreak havoc in their lives.

Symptoms of PMDD are generally similar to PMS, but tend to be much more severe. Additionally, women with PMDD can experience severe depression and anxiety. Treatment for PMDD includes antidepressants, anti-anxiety drugs and hormone therapy. If you suspect you have PMDD, the condition can be managed. This book will help you, but because your symptoms are so severe, it is

3

essential that you consult your doctor and get the treatment, support and help you need to get your life back on track.

PMS can also aggravate other health conditions you may have, such as allergies, asthma, irritable bowel syndrome and depression – or make them harder to deal with. This is called 'premenstrual magnification' (PMM) and is defined as an underlying health problem that you have all month long, and that gets worse 7 to 14 days before your period.

It's not just a 'woman thing'

Though you may be cursing every male you know when you are suffering from PMS, recent evidence has shown that men may actually suffer from PMS too. Irritable male syndrome, or IMS, produces symptoms that are very similar to those caused by PMS. Between 30 and 50 per cent of men are thought to suffer regularly from male PMS symptoms including depression, fatigue, headaches, back pain and hot flushes. Like PMS, IMS is thought to be triggered by fluctuations in hormones, specifically testosterone, the male sex hormone. This is often brought on by episodes of stress and by high-fat diets. In order to get IMS relief, stress reduction and a low-fat, balanced diet is recommended.

The causes of PMS

Even though PMS is now a recognized medical condition, it is still frequently misunderstood and misdiagnosed by doctors. This is probably because the symptoms and possible causes vary so widely from woman to woman. Despite all the uncertainty, however, PMS is definitely linked to your menstrual cycle, as research shows that if a woman is pregnant or has her ovaries removed, her symptoms typically disappear.

Here are some of the most common explanations[2] for PMS you may read about or hear from your doctor:

Hormonal imbalances

Many experts believe that PMS is caused by hormonal fluctuations and imbalances, and there are plenty of studies to back this up. It is thought that an imbalance in levels of the female sex hormones, progesterone and oestrogen, are most likely to trigger symptoms. Progesterone and oestrogen are produced in the ovaries, and while

4

oestrogen produces energy, progesterone acts as a balancer and a calmer. If the balance between progesterone and oestrogen in your body is right, you feel good, but if the balance is upset this can cause PMS. It is possible that your PMS could be due to any of the following hormonal shifts involving progesterone and oestrogen:

Oestrogen levels that are too high

Oestrogen boosts energy and well-being, but higher than normal amounts of this hormone may trigger bloating, weight gain and breast tenderness associated with PMS as well as anxiety, depression, insomnia and fatigue. Too much oestrogen can also cause blood sugar imbalances and magnesium deficiency, which can contribute to sugar cravings and mood swings. Higher than normal levels of oestrogen can be caused by a poor diet, stress, too much body fat (fatty tissue attracts oestrogen), oral contraceptives and liver dysfunction (the liver deactivates old oestrogen once it has done its job, so if the organ is not working well, oestrogen levels can build up). We are constantly exposed to man-made oestrogens through pesticides, plastics, pollution, hormone-laden meats and other environmental toxins – and all these can increase oestrogen levels in your body.

Low levels of oestrogen/serotonin

Although too much oestrogen is not good news, too little isn't either. This is because oestrogen plays a role in stimulating the brain cells that respond to the 'feel-good' hormone serotonin which has a mood-enhancing effect. A lack of serotonin can cause depression, irritability, migraines, hot flushes and vaginal dryness. Low levels of oestrogen/serotonin may be caused by a poor diet, stress and smoking among other things.

Low levels of progesterone

Progesterone counterbalances oestrogen, so if your progesterone levels are too low, symptoms of oestrogen excess may appear, even if oestrogen levels are normal. Progesterone is a natural diuretic that helps the body break down fat and use it for energy. It also keeps blood sugar levels stable, has an antidepressant effect, and helps you sleep better. If progesterone levels are too low, you may experience the opposite effect and have symptoms of PMS.

A lack of progesterone may be caused by too much oestrogen or lack of ovulation as, after ovulation, the old discarded follicle of the egg manufactures progesterone once the egg begins its journey to the fallopian tubes. A poor diet can also deplete progesterone levels, as too much saturated fat interferes with the manufacture of progesterone, as does a deficiency in antioxidants. Stress can also lower progesterone levels because stress releases large amounts of stress hormones, such as cortisol, adrenaline and androgen; these are antagonistic to progesterone.

Other explanations for PMS

PMS runs in the family

Unfortunately, if your mother, aunt or sister have PMS, you are more likely to have it yourself as research suggests PMS may be an inherited problem.

Birth control pills

For some women the pill cuts out PMS, but for others it can make the situation worse, depending on whether it balances your hormones or triggers an imbalance.

Nutritional deficiencies[3]

What you eat or don't eat can make PMS worse, especially if your diet is high in caffeine, saturated fat, alcohol, sugar and salt. Not getting enough essential nutrients can be caused by a poor diet, stress or pollution when the body uses up more nutrients than normal to protect itself. Research has linked deficiencies in essential fatty acids, Vitamin B6, calcium and magnesium to PMS.

Stress

Some experts[4] believe that stress may play a role in triggering or making symptoms of PMS worse. This is because stress affects the functioning of the adrenal glands, which produce hormones to regulate water balance, appetite and mood. The stress can be both emotional and physical.

All about you

Other possible causes of PMS include lack of exercise, poor functioning of the thyroid gland, food allergies, mercury fillings and yeast overgrowth, but even though there are a number of commonly accepted explanations, the exact cause of PMS remains unknown. The conclusion that many experts come to is that it may not be the hormones themselves, or even lifestyle factors, that trigger PMS, but a woman's unique response to these hormones and lifestyle factors. It seems that both you, and the unique way that your body copes with the stresses demanded of it, are key when it comes to understanding the reason for your PMS.

Risk factors for PMS

Certain factors are thought to increase your risk of PMS:

- your mother, sister, aunt or grandmother has (or had) it;
- you have children – PMS tends to get worse with each child you have;
- you are in your thirties or forties – PMS tends to hit hardest in these decades;
- you had trouble tolerating the contraceptive control pill or have recently stopped taking the pill;
- you don't exercise;
- you have a stressful lifestyle;
- you have an unhealthy diet;
- your weight fluctuates.

Have I got PMS?

Research shows that up to 85–90 per cent of women experience PMS in their reproductive years and a large number of these women find that it interferes with everyday life. So if you think you have PMS, you are certainly not alone. Bear in mind, though, that certain well-known symptoms of PMS may quite possibly be signs of another condition. For example, it is easy to confuse your depression over a failed relationship or job loss with the depression of PMS; or your backache and craving for sweets to PMS, when they may actually point to bad posture and hypoglycaemia. If symptoms are causing you distress, it is always a good idea to have a check-up with your doctor to rule out other possible physical and psychological causes. Remember there are always two hallmarks of PMS to look out for:

1 the symptoms appear up to 14 days before the onset of your period;
2 the symptoms clear up once your period begins, or a couple of days into it.

In other words, if your symptoms appear at other times in your cycle, the chances are that you are confusing PMS with another condition.

Charting your symptoms

PMS is a sneaky set of symptoms that can be hard to pin down. That is why it is important to start charting your symptoms to ensure that you do not confuse them with other conditions. Many other conditions may have PMS-like symptoms, but don't forget that there is an important difference: PMS only occurs in the run-up to your period, whereas your non-PMS-related conditions occur at other times of the month.

To make sure it is PMS you are suffering from, record your symptoms through a typical month and for one or two months after. This way, you can find out if there is a relationship between your symptoms and your menstrual cycle. If it is PMS, your symptoms will cluster in the two weeks before your period starts. If it isn't PMS, symptoms will appear at other times of the month.

As you begin charting your symptoms, do bear in mind that your menstrual cycles are never absolutely regular. A regular cycle is said to last 28 days, although any cycle from 23 to 35 days is typical. Your cycle begins on the first day of your period; ovulation occurs between 10 and 14 days before your period starts. The following box is only a rough guide to what typically happens during a menstrual cycle, and because everyone is different you may have a shorter or a longer cycle – or it may be different every month.

Time of the month

Your menstrual cycle is controlled by a complicated interaction between the pituitary gland and the ovaries and the female sex hormones – progesterone and oestrogen. During each cycle your hormones, in particular oestrogen and progesterone, will peak and surge over an average of 28 days.

In the first half of the menstrual cycle, progesterone levels stay low, but levels of oestrogen rise and make the lining of the uterus grow and thicken. In response to follicle-stimulating hormone, an egg (ovum) in one of the ovaries starts to mature. Oestrogen levels peak at about day 14 of a typical 28-day cycle, and in response to a surge of luteinizing hormone, the egg leaves the ovary. This is called ovulation.

In the second half of the menstrual cycle, the egg begins to travel through the fallopian tube to the uterus. Progesterone levels now begin to rise and help to prepare the uterine lining for pregnancy. Oestrogen also works alongside progesterone to make preparations for a possible pregnancy. On or near day 23, the levels of both progesterone and oestrogen reach an all-time high. If the egg becomes fertilized by a sperm cell and attaches itself to the uterine wall, the woman becomes pregnant. If the egg is not fertilized, however, the egg dissolves or is absorbed into the body. Oestrogen and progesterone levels drop sharply, causing the thickened lining of the uterus to break down and shed itself about five days later during the menstrual period.

When you look at the menstrual cycle, it is easy to see what a central role hormones play. Before, during and after your period, hormones can shift wildly, causing mood swings, crying spells and irritability. These symptoms have a biological basis and there are ways you can help yourself to deal with them.

It is a good idea to get into the habit of charting your symptoms every day for two to three months. Don't just write down your physical symptoms (for example, bloating or headaches), write down your *emotional* symptoms as well (for example, feeling tearful or moody). The best time to write things down is last thing at night when you have a chance to reflect on your day. Charting your symptoms is not just about

9

diagnosing PMS – it is also about self-awareness and becoming more attuned to how PMS affects your life and your behaviour. Some women even find that self-monitoring is an effective treatment in itself because they reach a better understanding of their body and see their symptoms in perspective: a few days of problems that have a physical cause, and once they have homed in on those problems, they can find ways to both prepare for them (and warn partners, friends and colleagues if need be) and treat them.

OK, I've got PMS. Now what?

You may not be able to change your age or the fact that you have kids or a hectic lifestyle, but there are things you can do about PMS. The good news is that PMS isn't all in your mind and researchers[5] have found that making positive changes in your lifestyle can make a big difference in the symptoms you experience and how severe they are. You may at this stage have already decided to try a self-help approach, but first it still might be a good idea to visit your doctor just once so that PMS can be confirmed and any more serious condition can be ruled out.

In the next chapter we'll explore what your doctor might offer you if PMS is diagnosed, and then in the chapters that follow we'll explore the range of self-help options available.

2

What your doctor might offer you

In most cases you may find that your doctor recommends self-help treatments as the first resort. These would include changes in diet and exercise routine, and possibly nutritional supplements. Forgetting for a moment the self-help remedies that your doctor would probably suggest, and which are discussed in the rest of this book, let's take a very brief look at hormonal treatments that your doctor might offer you if PMS is diagnosed and symptoms are severe.

Treatment options

The pill

The contraceptive pill is often recommended because it levels out naturally occurring peaks and slumps in your monthly cycle and protects you from swings towards too much or too little progesterone and oestrogen. The pill can be an effective treatment for some women, but it must be pointed out that a small number of women find that they continue to suffer symptoms when on the pill. The pill can also have a number of unpleasant side-effects include bloating and mood swings, and women who have never suffered from PMS may find that they experience PMS for the first time when coming off the pill.

Danazol

This is a powerful hormonal drug used for the treatment of endometriosis, breast pain, heavy bleeding, and other menstrual problems. It commonly produces disturbing side-effects such as nausea, swollen feet/ankles, weight gain, acne/oily skin, and excess body hair. Because of these side-effects, other treatments should be tried first.

Progesterone

One of the medical treatments for women with severe and incapacitating PMS is progesterone therapy. Progesterone, as we have seen, is the menstrual-cycle hormone that is produced after

11

ovulation and that drops to a low level before menstruation begins. Some researchers think that PMS is caused either by a deficiency in progesterone, by the drop in progesterone, or by a lower ratio of progesterone to oestrogen.

Two kinds of progesterone are used in the treatment of PMS: 'natural' and synthetic. 'Natural' progesterone is derived from yams or soya beans and is chemically similar to the progesterone produced by your body. It is given in rectal or vaginal suppositories or as an injection because it cannot be absorbed when taken by mouth. You can find out more about natural progesterone in Chapter 6. The synthetic progesterone (a drug that acts like progesterone in the body) is called progestogen. These can be taken as tablets. The most commonly prescribed progestogen for PMS is called Duphaston.

Progestogens can cause side-effects such as itchy skin; worsening of certain types of migraine and epilepsy; acne; weight gain; digestive disorders; depression; irregular periods; changes in sex drive; breast discomfort; insomnia; hair loss; excess hair growth; and worsening of premenstrual symptoms. Progestogens are taken a few days before premenstrual symptoms are expected and are stopped when menstruation begins. The doses should be tailored to suit the individual woman.

Hormone Replacement Therapy (HRT)

Some researchers think that a lack of oestrogen (rather than progesterone) is the problem behind PMS. Studies have found that some women benefit from hormone replacement therapy, either in the form of oestrogen implants or patches, combined with seven days a month of oral progestogen. The oestrogen stops ovulation, and the progestogen causes a monthly bleed and protects you from endometrial cancer. This treatment is only for women with severe PMS and requires close supervision by a gynaecologist. There are increased risks of breast cancer and blood clots with long-term use of HRT.

Antidepressants

Recent studies have shown that the more modern antidepressants, for example the selective serotonin re-uptake inhibitors (SSRIs), such as Prozac, can help with the emotional symptoms of PMS, particularly in women who also have an underlying depressive illness. However, unless depression is the only severe symptom of PMS you suffer, antidepressants are unlikely to be of much benefit.

Antiprostaglandins

Prostaglandins are substances produced by your body and they are responsible for producing pain and inflammation. Antiprostaglandin drugs, which include aspirin and Nurofen, may be prescribed to relieve physical symptoms of PMS, such as cramps, headaches, bloating, nausea and breast pain.

Diuretics

These are used for weight gain associated with bloating and swelling, but not for other symptoms. They are an artificial way of making your kidneys excrete more fluid, but you run the risk of excreting too much potassium. There are side-effects, and they should not be taken long term.

Treatment options to avoid

Anti-anxiety drugs are sometimes used to provide temporary relief from anxiety that limits your ability to cope with everyday life. They promote relaxation by reducing nerve activity in the brain. The trouble with anti-anxiety drugs is that they can be addictive and also trigger depression, so if your doctor suggests these you might want to ask for something else.

Another treatment option to be especially wary of is hysterectomy. A hysterectomy can often make PMS worse as unless the ovaries are removed, the cycle continues. Provera and Depo-Provera tablets or injections are also not helpful as they can cause depression. (Progesterone does not come in tablet form.) Electroconvulsive therapy (ECT) is a radical and controversial treatment for PMS that not only has serious and damaging long-term consequences, but has been shown to offer no benefits.

What you can do for yourself

Although PMS remains a puzzle, it is possible to avoid the drug option if your symptoms are not severe. You can examine what is known about PMS, and from that create a self-help plan of action tailored to your needs. You really do not have to suffer any longer and put your life on hold for one or two weeks every month. There is so much you can do to help yourself.[6] Used singly or in combination, the simple changes that are recommended in the following chapters can help you decrease or eliminate many, if not all, of your symptoms. Finally, you can start living life to the full, every single day.

3

Eat to beat PMS

One of the most effective ways to treat PMS isn't through medication or hormone therapy, but through a healthy diet that can balance your hormones and blood sugar levels. You may even find that what you thought was PMS disappears when you start eating a healthy diet.

Most experts[7] agree that the first line of treatment for PMS should be dietary. Links have been found between the food you eat and symptoms of PMS. The condition of PMS is associated with both hormonal and blood sugar imbalance and deficiencies of certain nutrients, so you may just find that changing your diet is the key to beating your symptoms. This is because imbalances of blood sugar or stress hormones or nutritional deficiencies can often trigger symptoms that are indistinguishable from PMS.

It is clear that some foods contribute to hormone imbalance while others restore that balance, but how do you eat to beat PMS? Fortunately, the dietary guidelines for beating PMS are in line with basic nutritional requirements for a healthy mind and body. Below you'll find 12 basic principles of healthy eating, along with the reasons they can help you beat PMS.

Twelve basic principles of healthy eating

1 Drink more water

Headaches, fatigue, dizziness and stomach upsets are all symptoms of PMS, but they can also be symptoms of dehydration.

Your body is two-thirds water, and water intake and distribution is vital for hormonal function. You need to drink plenty of water to keep your hormonal systems working at their best. Water also keeps your skin healthy and your eyes sparkling. It delivers nutrients to your organs and helps your body eliminate waste and toxins. Without water, you can feel dizzy, tired and bloated – not helpful when you are dealing with PMS! So drink plenty of fresh water, at least six to eight glasses a day. One way to make sure you are drinking enough fluids is to fill a bottle with your targeted amount of water and drink it throughout the day. Take it with you in the car or to work or keep it nearby. If the container is empty by bedtime, you've achieved your goal.

2 Eat at least five portions of fruit and vegetables each day

If you have PMS, vegetables and most fruits are essential. The vitamins and minerals and other nutrients they contain help balance fluctuating hormone levels and ease PMS, and they can also keep your bones strong, boost your immune system, calm the nervous system, ease depression and aid digestion because of their fibre content. For more information about essential nutrients for PMS, most of which are found in fruits and vegetables, read Chapter 4.

3 Eat regular snacks to balance your blood sugar

Irritability, mood swings, forgetfulness, anxiety, confusion, problems with concentration, feeling tearful, food cravings, fatigue and headaches are all symptoms of PMS. They are also symptoms of fluctuating blood sugar levels. Balancing blood sugar levels is one of the best treatments for PMS. This is because it is thought that changes in your body chemistry in the week before your period make your body much more sensitive to insulin, the hormone that helps to stabilize glucose levels in your body. Many women end up with lower than usual levels of blood glucose and that's why you feel fed up, irritable and moody and get food cravings – usually for sweet foods.

If your blood sugar levels are not stable, or are fluctuating wildly, this can trigger the production of adrenaline. Adrenaline is a stress hormone that can block the uptake of progesterone in your body and triggers symptoms of PMS. If blood sugar levels are stable, however, progesterone is released and symptoms are not triggered. The blood sugar-level theory explains why women with PMS may have similar amounts of progesterone and oestrogen to women who do not have PMS. Their bodies release enough progesterone, but cannot make use of it because of fluctuating blood sugar levels.

The best way to keep your blood sugar levels stable is to eat regular healthy snacks. Blood sugar levels drop sharply when you go for long periods without meals. Eating five or six meals and snacks a day is thought to be one of the best ways to combat PMS irritability, aggression, fatigue, dizziness, clumsiness and headaches. All these symptoms are associated with the low blood sugar that often occurs in the premenstrual phase. The best way to plan your meals is to eat a good breakfast followed by a mid-morning snack, lunch, a mid-afternoon snack and supper. That way you'll never get too hungry and your blood sugar levels remain stable. It is not a good idea to skip meals or fast. The aim is to keep blood sugar stable with a regular supply of nutrient-rich food, so do not go for more than a few hours without a meal or a snack.

4 Eat a little protein with each meal

Protein helps to balance your blood sugar, preventing the dips and highs in blood sugar that can bring about many PMS symptoms. Protein also gives your body an even supply of the amino acids it needs to build and repair cells and manufacture hormones and brain chemicals. Since your body cannot store protein, as it does with carbohydrates and fat, you need a constant supply. That is why you need to eat small portions of good-quality protein with every meal. Good-quality protein comes in the form of wholegrains, vegetables, nuts and seeds, low-fat dairy products, soya products, eggs, lean meat and fish. You will find that incorporating protein in your meals is actually quite simple: for breakfast you might have toast with peanut butter, or cereal with milk; for lunch you might have chilli with beans or wholewheat pitta bread with hummus; and for dinner you could have rice with beans or wholemeal pasta with chicken. For snacks you could have a banana with a handful of nuts and seeds.

5 Eat the right carbohydrates

Another way to keep your blood sugar levels steady, apart from regular snacks and eating protein with each meal, is to eat complex, low glycaemic (GI) carbohydrates instead of simple carbohydrates.

Low GI carbohydrates take longer to convert to glucose, giving you sustained energy and hormone balance. Potatoes, brown pasta, vegetables, dried fruit and wholemeal breads are typical sources of complex carbohydrates. Simple sugars found in refined foods, sweets, cakes, biscuits, and some fruits, tend to raise blood sugar too quickly. A quick way to work out the GI of a particular food without resorting to charts is to think about how refined it is. If it is highly refined – that is, it has lots of sugar, salt, additives and preservatives – it is going to make symptoms of PMS worse. The less refined it is – for example, brown rice, wholegrains and vegetables – the more it is going to lower blood sugar. Choose foods that are as close as possible to their raw or natural state and base your diet on foods that are rich in fibre. The glycaemic index is helpful if you have PMS, but it should not be the only dietary guideline on which to base your food choices. Remember too that when you are eating your carbohydrates (which should consist of around 40–50 per cent of your diet) you need to combine them with a little protein. For example, a baked potato has a high GI, but if you eat it with some tuna or low-fat cottage cheese it has a stabilizing effect on blood sugar.

6 Eat plenty of fibre

Fibre, like protein, is important for PMS because it slows down the release of blood sugar, thus helping to maintain blood-sugar balance. It also keeps your digestion healthy, allowing waste to pass through at a steady rate – which ensures less bloating and prevents the build-up of hormones and toxins being reabsorbed into the bloodstream. Ideally you should aim to eat around 30 g to 50 g of fibre daily. This is not a great amount, but you still need to drink plenty of fluid to ensure that it passes through your digestive system. You can get your fibre in wholegrain foods, nuts, seeds, fruits and vegetables. As a rough guide, an apple has around 2 g of fibre and an orange 3 g. Eat your five portions of fruit and vegetables a day and you are halfway there.

7 Make sure you get enough essential fatty acids (EFAs)

If you are not eating enough fat, or are eating too much of the wrong kind of fat, you will not be getting enough essential fatty acids (EFAs) in your diet and this could trigger symptoms of PMS.

Your body needs certain essential fats, including omega 3 fatty acid and omega 6 fatty acid (gamma linolenic acid), to regulate hormone function. If you are eating enough essential fatty acids in your diet, not only will your skin, hair and nails feel healthy and strong, but PMS symptoms will also ease. This is because EFAs satisfy your hunger, slow down the entry of carbohydrates, and keep blood sugar levels lower. Without the right amount of EFAs, your body cannot manufacture many important substances including ovarian hormones. Essential fats can also help to reduce swelling and inflammation of the body – if you are prone to swollen, tender breasts and abdomen due to PMS. And healthy skin that's spot-free is encouraged by EFAs, so they really are good for you in so many ways.

As a guideline, around 20–25 per cent of your diet should come from good fat, such as omega 3 and 6 fatty acids found in nuts, seeds, olive oil and oily fish (mackerel, salmon, herrings and sardines). Saturated animal fats found in red meat, cakes, pastries and trans-fatty acids found in many commercial foods should be avoided because they are low in nutrients and rich in substances that can increase your risk of obesity and heart disease. Excellent sources of omega 6 include evening primrose oil, blackcurrant oil and borage seed oil. You can also increase your intake of linolenic acid, the substance your body uses to manufacture gamma linolenic acid, by including light vegetable oils like safflower, corn, sunflower or soya oil in your diet. Perhaps the simplest solution, however, is to take flaxseed or hempseed oil, which contains both linolenic acid and omega 3 acids.

In a nutshell (so to speak!), aim to eat fish at least twice a week, especially coldwater fish like herring, salmon, mackerel and tuna. You should also eat nuts and seeds (linseed, sunflower, pumpkin, sesame, hemp, almonds, cashews, walnuts) daily, maybe as a snack between meals. Finally, you can take flax oil daily by the tablespoon or in salad dressings, or you could add hempseed oil to smoothies.

8 Eat phytoestrogens

Phytoestrogens are health-boosting substances found in plants that can have balancing effects on oestrogen, increasing levels when they are low and decreasing them when they are too high. As such they can be very helpful in treating PMS.

Phytoestrogens occur naturally in soya, linseeds, wheat, rice, oats, barley, carrots, potatoes, apples, cherries, plums and parsley, and in herbs such as sage, hops and liquorice. Vegetables oils such as olive, soya, flaxseed, groundnut and coconut oils may also be high in phytoestrogens.

The best way to increase the amount of phytoestrogens is to eat a diet rich in plant foods – vegetables, fruit and wholegrains. Try also to eat a couple of servings of soya-based foods a week. Soya beans are easy to cook and delicious when added to salads, soups or bakes. Soya yogurts or milk added to carbohydrates have a refreshing and pleasant taste. Tofu in thin slices can be added to stir fries, or whizzed in a blended smoothie; tempeh is great grilled in a sandwich. Start getting used to buying and eating soya-based products. Not only do they taste good, they are good for you too.

9 Ditch the salt

If you have problems with PMS water retention, bloating, weight gain or breast swelling, they could be the result of too much salt in your diet.

The more salt you eat, the more your body holds on to water in your tissues to avoid dehydration. So, if you tend to retain water, the more salt (sodium) you eat, the worse your problem gets. Fluid retention can raise blood pressure as well. You cannot avoid salt altogether, but you can take steps to reduce your sodium intake. Instead of salt, try using herbs, spices, lemon juice, wine or ginger to flavour your food. Have fun experimenting with spices and alternatives until you find those that you like best.

Get into the habit of checking the salt content of foods you eat. There are hidden salts in most of the foods we buy and eat today, especially ones that have chemicals and additives and preservatives in them. Some foods claim to be reduced salt or low salt, but this can be confusing as most manufacturers talk about sodium. To find out how much salt there is in the food you buy, multiply the sodium content by 2.5. Aim for less than 5 g a day. In time you will get used to a less salty diet and start to really taste food again, free from the overpowering taste of salt.

10 Pass on the sugar

We touched on this earlier with the 'eat the right carbohydrate' principle, but it is so important it can be stressed again.

Although PMS is a complicated disorder, there is one thing everyone seems to agree on: sugar makes it worse. Sugar stimulates the production of too much insulin which causes your blood sugar levels to plummet. If your blood sugar levels are low, you feel edgy and tired and are likely to crave more sugar – which gives you a brief high followed by a big slump. It is a vicious circle that can leave you feeling irritable throughout the PMS phase. Sugar can also overwork the liver and make it unable to process oestrogen, effectively causing oestrogen levels to rise. Excess sugar also triggers the production of stress hormones, which have the undesirable effect of lowering progesterone. Finally, sugar also works against good nutrition and can deplete your body of nutrients.

The solution is simple: cut down on your sugar intake, especially in your PMS phase. If you feel your blood sugar level dipping, don't reach for chocolate or sugary foods that can drive up your blood sugar levels quickly – eat something containing complex carbohy-drates that can give you a steady release of sugar. Bear in mind that refined foods, like white bread, white rice, instant potato and cornflakes, can act like sugar in your system because they lack fibre. It is always best to stick with wholegrains and fresh fruits and vegetables and to eat some protein at the same time to keep your blood sugar levels from skyrocketing.

If you want to assess your sugar intake, you need to start checking food labels because sugar is a hidden ingredient in many foods, especially processed ones. It has many different names including the following: brown sugar, concentrated fruit juice, corn syrup, dextrose, fructose, glucose, honey, lactose, maltose, molasses, raw sugar and sucrose. You should also get rid of the sugar bowl and opt for fresh fruit rather than tinned fruit. Try the low-sugar versions of jams and jellies. Cinnamon, cardamom, ginger, nutmeg and other spices can also give a sweet flavour without adding sugar.

You may find it extremely hard to cut down on sugar at the time of the month you tend to crave it, but once you do manage to avoid it, and instead eat six wholesome, nutritious and healthy meals a day, you should find that your cravings recede. You may think that sugar is your friend when you feel low – but, believe me, it isn't. Do pass on the sugar.

11 Cut down on caffeine

Caffeine is a stimulant that increases sleeplessness, anxiety and tension, which are all parts of the PMS problem. It can be found in coffee, tea, soft drinks and chocolate and in some over-the-counter pain relievers. Even decaffeinated drinks contain some caffeine.

One study[8] of college-age women found severe PMS symptoms in 60 per cent of those who drank more than four cups of caffeinated drinks a day. We know that even tiny amounts will stimulate the release of adrenaline, which isn't good news if you have PMS. And coffee is metabolized slowly – even one cup or soft drink at dinner may stop you sleeping well. Coffee also causes your body to get rid of important nutrients, especially the B vitamins needed to fight PMS.

It is best to cut down on caffeine as much as possible, especially if you get PMS breast tenderness, but if you can't do that, at least cut down in the two weeks before your period. Just cutting back on your intake can make a positive difference. Aim for one or two caffeinated drinks a day at most.

If you are used to drinking more than two cups of coffee a day, or a couple of caffeine-containing beverages a day, it isn't a good idea to cut them out immediately. Caffeine narrows your blood vessels, and if you suddenly stop, your blood vessels will widen and you will get splitting headaches. Take it easy and cut back gradually. If you taper it off slowly, withdrawal symptoms such as headaches should not last more than two weeks. Start by limiting your intake to two or three cups of tea or coffee a day and start substituting a glass of water at the other times, supplemented with a slice of lemon to give it a sharper taste. Or try decaffeinated teas, coffees and soft drinks, or grain-based 'coffee' such as Postum or Caffix, or refreshing herbal teas. Or substitute diluted fresh pressed juices or smoothies; they are delicious, energy-boosting and good for you.

12 Limit alcohol consumption

Drinking alcohol will make your symptoms worse, especially in the two weeks before your period when your body is more sensitive to its effects. It interferes with hormonal function and the proper absorption of B vitamins and magnesium, which – as you will see in the next chapter – are essential for beating PMS.

Alcohol can also cause low blood sugar by blocking the body's ability to supply glucose when it is needed. And to top it all, alcohol is a depressant. The best strategy while you are trying to beat PMS is to avoid alcohol altogether, but if you do want to drink, do so as an occasional treat, drink only with a meal, and try to drink only when you are not feeling premenstrual. The rest of the time try non-alcoholic drinks like sparkling mineral water with a slice of lemon, fresh pressed juice diluted with spring water, or alcohol-free beer or wine. Once you have eliminated PMS, you can drink alcohol in moderation again. Try not to drink every night, but if you do, two glasses of wine is your absolute maximum.

Suggestions for vegetarians

It is important to make sure you get enough protein if you are a vegetarian. You need to replace animal protein with other food sources such as dairy products, pulses, legumes, nuts, seeds, grains and cereal for otherwise deficiencies in Vitamins B12 (almost only found in animal products, including meat and fish) and D, calcium and iron are likely to trigger nutritional and hormonal imbalance and make your PMS worse. Here are some suggestions to help you do this:

- If you are the only vegetarian in your household, make sure you substitute pulses, beans, wholegrain cereals, dairy products, tofu products or Quorn instead of just leaving the meat part out of the meal.
- Choose cereals fortified with vitamins, especially Vitamin B12. Try to eat a large portion of dark-green leafy vegetables every day and around a pint of whole or skimmed milk. If you are lactose intolerant, you can get your calcium in calcium-enriched soya yogurts and milks or nut milks.
- Eat dried fruits, pulses, green vegetables and wholegrains for fibre and iron. Cocoa powder and dark chocolate are good sources of iron too.
- Eat at least 30 g of pulses, nuts and seeds every day for protein and essential fatty acids (EFAs).
- Eat at least one serving of low-fat cheese or cottage cheese a day for protein and calcium – or a soya pattie or tofu portion.
- Eat a total of three to four eggs a week.
- Choose margarine or butter fortified with Vitamin D and E in a vegetarian spread. You can get Vitamin D from sunlight as well and Vitamin E from nuts and seeds.

If you are vegan, you may need expert advice from a doctor or nutritionist. The Vegan Society websites have plenty of useful information. Make sure you get enough protein and Vitamin B12. The American Diabetic Association states that soya protein has been shown to be nutritionally equivalent in protein value to animal protein. Nuts, seeds, grains, pulses and vegetables are other good sources of protein. Yeast extracts used as food flavourings are often high in Vitamin B12, but they are not high enough, and all vegans are advised to take a specific B12 supplement.

Give yourself a break

The 12 principles outlined above will help balance your blood sugar levels and your hormones, but as you incorporate them into your lifestyle, try not to set yourself up for failure and remember the 80/

20 rule. It is the indulgences or excesses that trigger symptoms, and as long as you are eating healthily most of the time – say 80 per cent – you can allow yourself the occasional indulgence. You don't have to give up chocolate, coffee or your snacks – you just need to eat them in moderation. No food should be completely banned in a PMS-beating diet, as the key to a healthy diet and happy life is variety.

4

Essential vitamins and minerals to beat PMS

If you are eating a healthy diet according to the guidelines given in the previous chapter, the chances are you are getting all the nutrients you need to balance your hormones; but there are certain nutrients that are so essential for hormonal balance that they do need special mention. Below you will find a list of food sources and recommended daily doses of essential vitamins and minerals to beat PMS.

The good guys

Vitamin A and beta-carotene (which comes from plant sources) function as immune-boosting antioxidants that can help keep your skin healthy and fight spots and pimples caused by PMS. Foods rich in Vitamin A include egg yolk, butter, milk and oily fish. Foods rich in beta-carotene include red, orange and green vegetables, sweet potatoes and carrots. The recommended dosage for treating PMS is 15,000 iu daily.

Vitamin B complex is essential for stabilizing blood sugar, easing mood swings, decreasing sugar cravings, improving sleep, and fighting fatigue and headaches. Vitamin B also helps the liver to deactivate and dispose of old oestrogen, which helps guard against oestrogen excess. In addition, Vitamin B complex supports adrenal function, which decreases sugar cravings and headaches. The vitamins in the B complex are typically found together in food, and include thiamin, niacin, biotin, riboflavin, pantothenic acid, Vitamin B6, PAPA, choline, inositol, Vitamin B12 and folic acid. Food sources include wholegrains, legumes, brewer's yeast, dairy produce, eggs, vegetables, fish, nuts, watermelon, avocado and seaweed. The recommended dosage for beating PMS is 50 mg to 100 mg daily of the Vitamin B complex.

Vitamin B6 is especially important for the regulation of mood, memory, water balance and sleep. Several studies[9] have shown that Vitamin B6 can reduce the discomfort associated with PMS and that there is a link between B6 deficiency and PMS. A lack of Vitamin B6 can ease irritability, depression, mood swings, breast tenderness, fatigue, sugar cravings, acne and water retention. B6 also plays a part in producing prostaglandins, substances that can help to maintain a healthy oestrogen/progesterone balance. The recommended daily dosage for helping to combat PMS is 50–220 mg.

Vitamin C functions as an anti-stress and immune-boosting antioxidant vitamin. It helps to fight fatigue, aches and pains, and sugar cravings, and it also lessens water retention, eases breast swelling, assists the liver in breaking down oestrogen and boosts the immune system. Food sources include all fruits and vegetables, especially sprouts, red peppers, citrus fruits and dark-green and yellow leafy vegetables. The recommended dosage for treating PMS is 500–1,000 mg a day.

Vitamin D is important for energy. Vitamin D-fortified margarine, eggs and oily fish are good sources, but it can also be produced in the skin if it is exposed to light. Vitamin D should not be taken in large doses – 100 iu is the recommended daily dose for easing PMS.

Vitamin E is a powerful antioxidant that boosts immunity. It can also improve the efficiency of insulin. Research[10] has shown it can help to ease breast tenderness. It may also relieve depression, insomnia and fatigue. Plant oils, including sunflower and corn and unrefined wholegrain cereals, are good food sources of Vitamin E. It can also be found in sweet potatoes, asparagus, broccoli, green leafy vegetables, green beans, nuts and seeds. The recommended dosage for treating PMS is 400 iu a day.

Boron is essential for the efficient functioning of calcium and magnesium (two minerals that are important for controlling PMS). It can help to ease mood swings, water retention, headaches, sugar cravings and other effects of calcium and magnesium deficiency. Food sources include fruits and vegetables, especially apples, peaches, pears, grapes, legumes and peanuts. The recommended dosage for treating PMS is 3–9 mg.

Calcium is essential for growth and the maintenance of healthy bones and teeth. It can also ease water retention, mood swings, headaches and pain. Studies[11] have found that calcium supplements can be extremely beneficial for those with PMS, although experts aren't sure why. It could be the result of its anti-inflammatory efforts and the role it plays in the production of serotonin, the body's 'feel-good' chemical. Dairy products, calcium-fortified soya milk, sardines, spinach, almonds and wholegrain cereals and bread are good sources of calcium. The recommended dosage for treating PMS is

400–700 mg. The best kind of calcium supplement to take is calcium citrate because it is easily absorbed.

Chromium is an important mineral for the control of blood sugar levels as it works with insulin to help the glucose, your body's fuel, get into the cells. It can help with weight gain, acne, blood sugar problems and cravings, irritability and fatigue. Food sources include liver, brewer's yeast, nuts and wholegrains. The recommended dosage for treating PMS is 200–400 mg of chromium picolinate, the most absorbable form of chromium.

Iodine is necessary for healthy thyroid function and regulation of metabolism and oestrogen levels. A deficiency can result in menstrual problems, oestrogen build-up and PMS fatigue. Food sources include seafood, kelp, saltwater fish, seaweed, sesame seeds, soya beans and garlic. The recommended daily dosage for iodine is 150 mg.

Iron is important for energy production. One of the most common causes of fatigue is iron levels falling too low, leading to anaemia. Good food sources include red meat, liver, eggs, spinach and pulses. The recommended daily dosage for iron is 15 mg.

Magnesium plays an essential role in the body's metabolic processes and works in conjunction with calcium to convert fat, carbohydrates and protein into energy and to regulate blood sugar and the heartbeat. Magnesium deficiency has been associated with PMS.[12] One study of magnesium levels and PMS showed a reduction in breast tenderness and bloating in 95 per cent of subjects. Magnesium can help to reduce water retention and ease headaches, mood swings, sugar cravings, fatigue and low energy. Food sources include wheat bran, wheatgerm, nuts, flour, dark-green leafy vegetables, dried apricots, fish and tofu. The recommended dosage for treating PMS is 200–600 mg. A deficiency in magnesium will affect calcium metabolism, so it is very important to balance your magnesium with your calcium intake.

Selenium is found in meat, fish (especially mackerel, herring and kippers) and wholemeal flour, and deficiency has been linked to period problems and infertility in women. The recommended daily dosage is 60–75 mcg.

Zinc helps to stimulate the immune system and control the inflammation of acne. It is a component of many of the body's hormones, including insulin, the sex hormones and thyroid hormones. Zinc deficiency can trigger oestrogen excess, the production of inflammation-causing prostaglandins, and suppress the action of progesterone. Food sources include seafood, liver, eggs, wholegrains, dried beans and peas. The recommended dosage for treating PMS is 25–50 mg.

In the 1980s, the amino acid DLPA was made available to treat pain and depression as it protects and strengthens your endorphins, or feel-good hormones. DLPA is a mixture of the essential amino acid L-phenylalanine and its mirror-image D-phenylalanine, found in most protein foods. DLPA also appears to influence certain chemicals in the brain that relate to pain sensation. If you do want to try DLPA, it is important that you consult your doctor first. DLPA should not be used if you are pregnant, or hoping to be.

Taking supplements

In an ideal world, we would be getting all the vitamins and minerals we need from our diet, but we *don't* live in an ideal world and there will be times when you feel stressed or rushed and unable to ensure optimum intake. That is why it is a good idea to start taking a good multivitamin and mineral supplement on a daily basis. A good supplement is never a substitute for a healthy diet, and it is essential to get as many nutrients as you can from your diet as it seems that your body absorbs nutrients better from food than from pills. But a good supplement can protect against nutritional deficiencies that might make PMS worse.

First thing in the morning is the best time to take your supplement. It is not really necessary to take different vitamins and minerals to help ward off PMS as most of what you need can be found in a good-quality vitamin and mineral supplement. The only possible exceptions are calcium and magnesium. Since most experts agree that calcium and magnesium are the most important nutrients for treating PMS, you might want to think about taking them separately, as no multivitamin will contain adequate amounts of these two essential nutrients for beating PMS. Do keep your supplement regime as simple as possible though, as the simpler it is the more likely you are to remember to take it.

Warning: Taking vitamin and mineral supplements in high doses can be dangerous, so make sure you consult your pharmacist or your doctor before self-prescribing.

Give it a try!

The importance of eating a nutrient-rich, healthy diet cannot be stressed enough when it comes to balancing your hormones and managing the symptoms of PMS. If your diet is poor, you are far more likely to suffer from PMS than if your diet is healthy. Many women do find that making positive alterations to their diet is the first and only change they need to make to reduce or eliminate their symptoms. Why not give it a try right now by planning a few days of healthy menus rich in the vitamins and minerals you need to beat PMS? You will find some samples below to get you thinking, cooking and eating along the right lines.

Sample PMS-busting recipes

Breakfast (with multivitamin and mineral supplement): Scrambled egg on wholegrain toast plus a glass of freshly pressed apple juice.
Snack: Glass of semi-skimmed organic milk and a piece of fresh fruit.
Lunch: Bowl of lentil soup and tuna, egg or hummus and salad sandwich.
Snack: Sesame snaps or oat and rice cakes, plus four dried apricots or dates.
Dinner: Chicken, tofu or bean burger with big mixed salad and small baked potato. Baked apples stuffed with raisins and served with low-fat vanilla yogurt.

Breakfast (with multivitamin and mineral supplement): Skimmed or soya milk porridge with chopped bananas and nuts, plus glass of freshly pressed apple juice.
Snack: Piece of fruit and small raisin biscuit.
Lunch: Avocado and salad sandwich on wholegrain bread plus small slice of chocolate cake.
Snack: Glass of milk plus fresh fruit.
Dinner: Wholemeal pasta with vegetables (onions, broccoli, sweetcorn, tomatoes) and topping of grated cheese, fresh fruit and nut salad.

Breakfast (with multivitamin and mineral supplement): Oat-based cereal with calcium-enriched skimmed milk, glass of freshly pressed apple juice.
Snack: Sesame seed biscuits.
Lunch: Broccoli soup, salmon fishcake, organic new potatoes, serving of spinach with scraping of butter.
Snack: Handful of nuts and raisins.
Dinner: Vegetable risotto, hot fruit with low-fat calcium-enriched yogurt.

Breakfast (with multivitamin and mineral supplement): Boiled free range egg, slice of stoneground wholemeal toast with a scraping of butter, and a glass of freshly pressed apple juice.
Snack: Piece of fruit and a small handful of fruit and nut mix.
Lunch: Chicken with green bean and sweetcorn salad or a bowl of carrot soup, plus pitta bread stuffed with chicken, or hummus and salad. Red fruit-based dessert – crumble tart or fresh fruit salad.
Snack: Vegetable sticks.
Dinner: Roasted vegetables (tomatoes, mushrooms, auber-gines, courgettes and new potatoes sprinkled with olive oil and roasted at 180°C for 20 mins), glass of red wine, dried fruit (figs, apricots, prunes and apple) topped with low-fat yogurt.

Breakfast (with multivitamin and mineral supplement): Fruit salad including a small banana, sprinkled with chopped nuts, glass of calcium-enriched soya milk, or nut milk or organic semi-skimmed milk.
Snack: Handful of mixed seeds and a piece of fruit.
Lunch: Greek salad, yogurt sprinkled with nuts.
Snack: Small packet of Twiglets, low-fat cottage cheese, piece of fruit.
Dinner: Grilled chicken or fish or tofu/bean burger and big green salad (cucumber, mixed leaves, spring onions, peppers, shredded crunchy cabbage) with new potatoes, garlic, lemon juice and hemp/pumpkin seed oil dressing, baked apple with cinnamon.

Breakfast (with multivitamin and mineral supplement): Wheat bran cereal topped with low-fat yogurt and a sprinkling of chopped nuts with soya milk, nut milk or semi-skimmed milk, glass of freshly pressed apple juice.

Snack: Dried apricots and crackers.
Lunch: Tofu with pasta salad and a slice of pumpkin and raisin bread.
Snack: A handful of mixed seeds and a piece of fruit.
Dinner: Dark-green leafy vegetables, new potatoes, beans and peas with fish. Stewed fruit with low-fat vanilla, strawberry or chocolate yogurt.

Breakfast (with multivitamin and mineral supplement, and magnesium): Wholemeal muffin with a teaspoonful of peanut butter and sliced banana, glass of milk and herbal tea.
Snack: Handful of mixed seeds.
Lunch: Baked potato filled with hummus or tuna and sweet-corn plus a bowl of salad and seasoned steamed vegetables, and a yogurt dessert.
Snack: Wholegrain rice cakes or oatcakes with organic low-fat cream cheese and a handful of grapes.
Dinner: Chicken and vegetable curry with steamed basmati rice and fruit-based dessert.

Once you have done the planning, why not give healthy eating a try for a couple of weeks and see how much fitter, slimmer and better you feel? Start today. You have got nothing to lose except PMS!

5

Get moving: PMS and exercise

You probably know already that regular physical activity provides enormous health benefits. Studies show that regular exercise:

- improves your chances of living longer;
- helps to lower high blood pressure (hypertension) and high cholesterol;
- improves your quality of life;
- helps to prevent osteoporosis (gradual loss of bone mass/strength);
- improves mobility and strength in later life;
- helps to protect you from developing certain cancers;
- reduces the risk of heart disease;
- helps prevent or control Type 2 diabetes (adult-onset diabetes);
- alleviates symptoms of depression and anxiety;
- helps with weight reduction and weight management.

And if that weren't enough, regular exercise also boosts your immunity, improves the way you look, and gives your sex drive a boost! By contrast, health studies that have monitored the well-being of large groups of people over many years clearly show that being inactive significantly *increases* the risk of being overweight (and obesity) and suffering from chronic diseases.

What exercise can do for your PMS

But did you know that regular exercise also helps to prevent or relieve PMS? Well, it can and it does. Research[13] has shown that regular, moderate exercise evokes hormonal responses from the body and can help with just about every symptom of PMS. Women who engage in moderate aerobic exercise at least three times a week have fewer symptoms than women who don't exercise. In fact, exercise may be one of the most effective, healthy and natural ways to combat your symptoms – especially those related to depression and tension, such as mood swings, fatigue, irritability and cramps.

For optimum results, most experts recommend at least 30 minutes of moderate exercise every day, especially during the premenstrual phase. This is because exercise can help to:

- *lower blood sugar levels by burning it as fuel*: The fitter you are, the lower your body fat and the better your insulin and glucose control. Fluctuating blood sugar levels, you may recall, can trigger or make worse PMS symptoms. Steady exercise for more than 20 minutes also allows your muscles to store more glucose, lowering your blood sugar levels even after you have stopped exercising.

- *reduce water retention*: Exercise gets your bodily fluids moving, and by so doing it relieves bloating and water retention. The excess water is sweated out.

- *encourage deep breathing*: Exercise encourages deep breathing, which improves circulation and brings oxygen to the tissues to prevent toxic substances building up that can trigger headaches, fatigue and pain.

- *beat stress*: Exercise is also a great stress-reliever, and don't we just need that when PMS strikes! Exerting yourself physically burns off stress hormones and gives your body an opportunity to release pent-up tension and anxiety.

- *ease aches and pains*: Exercise encourages good posture and strengthens muscles, and also takes pressure off organs and joints to relieve aches and pains.

- *boost your mood*: When you exercise, your body produces more endorphins, hormones that can increase your sense of well-being, relieve depression, ease mental tension, hostility and irritability and block pain. It has been suggested[14] that women with PMS may have only 20–50 per cent of the amount of endorphins circulating as compared to a woman without PMS. If this is the case, exercise is essential.

- *make you sleep better*: Exercise also improves the quality of your sleep – on the days you exercise, you tend to sleep better.

- *boost your energy levels*: One of the best things about exercising regularly is that you have more energy. You will feel less tired and more upbeat in general.

- *keep your hormones in balance*: Most important of all, it is thought that moderate exercise can suppress the overproduction of sex hormones and help to keep your hormones in balance.

With all these benefits, exercise simply has to be an essential part of your programme to beat PMS. Don't go crazy, though, and launch yourself into a vigorous exercise routine. Instead, begin slowly with mild exercise and then gradually build up, especially if you have not been active for a while. Walk instead of run, swim or cycle at an easy pace, and so on. Then once you feel stronger, you can increase the intensity and length of your workout, but, as before, make sure you do this gradually. If you are overweight or have a pre-existing medical condition, make sure you check with your doctor before beginning an exercise routine.

Your exercise prescription

Once you know it is safe for you to exercise, exercise safely! Use your common sense and listen to your body. Obviously when you first get going there will be some discomfort or even soreness after a session, but there should not be any pain, fainting, dizziness, shortness of breath or nausea. So don't overdo it. If something doesn't feel right, STOP immediately and talk to your doctor.

Be sure to wear loose comfortable clothing when exercising and check that your shoes offer the correct support. Drink plenty of water before, during and after your workout (even if you don't feel thirsty) and have light snacks on hand if you get a sudden dip in energy. Finally, pay attention to your breathing when you are exercising. Try to prevent it from becoming quick and shallow. You should breathe in deeply through your nose and out through your mouth.

To improve your health and quality of life you do not need to join a gym or run the marathon – you need just 30 minutes of activity per day. And you do not have to do the 30 minutes all at once – it can be spread out throughout the day and can include activities such as climbing stairs, a brisk walk, cleaning the house, walking while talking on the mobile, and so on. Any activity counts. You just need to get 30 minutes a day most days of the week. If you don't think you are getting your 30 minutes, find ways to reach this target: park farther away from work so you have got to walk; climb the stairs instead of using the lift; carry your shopping home; wash your car by hand, and mow the lawn. In the long run these simple changes can help to prevent health complications and make you feel better about yourself.

A good exercise routine that you can repeat daily, every other day or three times a week, starts with 5 to 10 minutes of gentle warm-up exercises to get your circulation going. Brisk walking, jumping or doing light stretches will get your body in the right mode for movement and help to prevent injuries. Your warm-up should be followed by moderately paced aerobic exercise that works the large muscles and elevates your heart rate for 20 to 30 minutes. The aim is to get your heart rate up to 60–75 per cent of its maximum capacity (220 minus your age). You should feel slightly out of breath, but not so much so that you cannot carry on a conversation. You don't have to join a class to do an aerobic workout. Anything that speeds up your heart rate and makes you breathe more deeply will qualify, including dancing, brisk walking or jogging, trampoline, playing sports, cycling and so on. Aerobic exercise is great for strengthening your heart, increasing lung capacity and burning up excess fat. This form of exercise is particularly helpful for PMS because it stimulates sweating, relieves muscle tension, burns stress hormones and stimulates endorphin release.

Fast walking is an ideal form of *aerobic exercise* if you suffer from PMS, but you may prefer jogging, cycling, an exercise class or swimming. Whatever you decide on, make sure you enjoy it. Studies show that 'exercise drop-outs' often punish themselves with exercise routines they don't enjoy. So if you hate jogging or swimming, don't do it! Find an exercise that you enjoy, so that you can stick with it. It doesn't have to be a traditional exercise or class – if dancing, rambling, horse riding or boxing are things you enjoy, make them part of your exercise routine. You may also want to ask your partner or a friend to exercise with you. When you exercise with other people, you are more likely to continue because you can motivate one another, and it is tougher to break a commitment to exercise if you are doing it with someone else. And, finally, if you *do* skip a workout, don't let it derail your exercise prescription. If you are working out five times a week for 30 minutes, giving yourself a day or two off now and again is not going to undo the good you've done.

In addition to your aerobic exercise, you will also need to include some *strength-bearing activities* two or three times a week for 10 to 15 minutes. The more muscle you have, the more calories you burn – and the better your blood sugar balance will be, even when you are not exercising. Good muscle tone will make you look fitter as well as protecting your joints from stress. Weight lifting, swimming, leg lifts, push-ups and isometric exercises (i.e. placing your palms together and pushing) are all examples of strength-bearing exercises.

Stretching exercises are something you need to do every day for 5 to 10 minutes to increase your overall flexibility and prevent injury. Stretching is also a great way to ease muscle pain and increase relaxation – all of which are helpful for PMS. Stretching should always be done slowly and carefully, and when you assume a stretching position you should only stretch as far as is comfortable. Do not bound, simply hold the stretch for 30 or so seconds, and towards the end of the time try to stretch just a little further, then slowly release.

Finally, don't forget to *cool down* for 5 to 10 minutes at the end of your exercise session. A 'cool down' is a bit like a 'warm-up', but this time you want to 'rev down' your body – not rev it up. Think of yourself as an athlete. You need to walk or gently jog along the track for a bit before you can stop completely.

Yoga and PMS

One of the best forms of exercise for PMS relief is yoga. Since PMS is made worse by stress, tension and upset, the calming, restorative effects of yoga may do much to ease your symptoms.

Yoga, a Sanskrit word meaning 'union', originated in India more than 5,000 years ago. The practice of yoga is designed to quieten the mind by teaching you how to pay attention to your breathing and to the movement or stillness of your body. Yoga[15] postures re-establish structural integrity by stretching and strengthening muscles, expanding the natural range of motion, massaging internal organs, relaxing nerves, increasing blood circulation and encouraging blood sugar and hormone balance. And, because yoga focuses and calms the mind, it can help to ease feelings of anxiety, fatigue and depression and prevent or alleviate many stress-related conditions.

The most popular form of yoga in the West is called Hatha yoga, which focuses on the mind–body balance, using physical postures, breathing techniques and meditation to restore the *prana*, which is the life energy or vital force that flows through every living being. To learn more about yoga, you may want to find a good instructor, but if there just aren't enough hours in the day, you will find below some simple yoga exercises to do by yourself at home.

Generally, you need to hold the posture for between 20 seconds and two minutes, often in conjunction with deep breathing exercises. The deep breathing increases oxygenation of body tissues and encourages relaxation. Even if you practise yoga for as little as five minutes every morning or evening, you can still experience the benefits.

Yoga exercises

Energizing breath

When you are feeling stressed, your breathing gets more shallow and rapid than usual, and you breathe from your chest. Your lungs are not fully expanded and so your body is rarely fully oxygenated. Just by taking a few deep breaths you can feel more relaxed. Try the following exercise in order to become a 'lung breather' rather than a 'chest breather'.

Place one hand on your chest and the other on your abdomen. When you take a deep breath in, the hand on the abdomen should rise higher than the one on the chest. This ensures that the diaphragm is pulling air into the bases of the lungs.

After exhaling through the mouth, take a slow deep breath in through your nose, imagining that you are sucking in all the air in the room, and hold it for a count of 7 (or as long as you are able, not exceeding 7).

Slowly exhale through your mouth for a count of 8. As air is released with relaxation, gently contract your abdominal muscles to completely evacuate the remaining air from the lungs.

Repeat the cycle four more times for a total of five deep breaths, completely filling and emptying your lungs each time.

Mountain pose

This yoga pose teaches correct posture and is the basis for all other standing poses. Stand with your feet together so your big toes are touching and your heels are slightly apart. Let your arms relax by your sides. Spread and lengthen your toes, make sure your kneecaps are facing forward, and keep your pelvis balanced by your legs. Now lengthen your spine by stretching from your inner legs from heel to groin. Continue to lengthen upwards, opening your chest. Drop your shoulders and lengthen the back of your neck. Hold this pose for one minute.

Sideways stretch

Stand straight with your legs three feet apart, your toes facing forwards. Inhale and lift your right arm in the air. As you exhale, gently bend over to the left side, sliding your hand down your left leg. Don't strain, just go as far as you can with ease. Breathing normally, hold the position for a count of 5 or 10 if you feel strong enough. Inhale and return slowly to an upright position. Exhale and slowly lower your arm and relax. Repeat the other side.

The cat

Assume a hands and knees position as if you were a cat, weight distributed evenly between your palms and your knees, fingers pointing forwards. As you slowly inhale, pull your stomach muscles tight and curve your back towards the ceiling, like a cat that is arching its back. Tuck your chin into your chest to complete the cat-like pose and hold for 5 counts. Then relax the spine and bring your head back to its normal position as you slowly exhale. Continue exhaling as you reverse the arch of your spine, pulling your head back towards your upper back and swaying your back just a little. Begin inhaling again as your head, neck and spine move back to a starting position. Continue inhaling as you repeat the exercise, first arching like a cat, then exhaling as you pull the head, neck and spine backwards. Do the exercise slowly and never rush.

Forwards and backwards bend

Do your energizing breath and your mountain pose. Inhale and slowly stretch your arms above your head. Exhale slowly through your nose as you bend forwards, keeping your back flat and legs straight until you reach your maximum without straining. Stay there for a count of 5 or 10, breathing normally. You may not be able to reach far to start with, but one day your chin will be on your shin if you keep practising! Inhale and come up slowly into an upright position, hands stretched above your head. Bend backwards, looking at your thumbs, exhaling in the maximum position. Breathing normally, hold for a count of 5, inhale, and return to upright. Exhale, lower your arms, and relax. Repeat.

Rishis posture

Do your energizing breath and mountain posture. Inhale and gently stretch your arms into the air. As you exhale, bend forwards slowly and, with your legs straight and back flat, grasp your left leg with your right hand. Don't strain – just grasp wherever is comfortable. Slowly lift your left arm and turn your body so that you are facing your left hand. Hold for a count of 5 or 10. Then slowly lower your arm and relax forwards, clasping your legs and gently pulling your body towards them. Inhale and, as you exhale, repeat the movement on the other side, raising your right arm. Relax forwards, clasping both legs and drawing your body inwards. Inhale and return to upright, stretching your arms above your head. Put your hands on your waist, with thumbs in front and fingers behind. Now gently bend back, exhaling as you reach maximum bend. Hold for 5. Inhale and return to upright. Exhale. Relax and repeat.

The child's pose

This is a good exercise to do at the end of a yoga session to ease your body into a totally relaxed state. Tuck your legs underneath you as you sit on a mat with your heels directly underneath your bottom and your knees pointing forwards. Pull your knees apart about 10 inches while keeping your toes together, forming a V with your thighs. Roll your upper body forward to the floor with your arms extended loosely in front of you. Your forehead should touch the floor if possible. You can separate your knees to do this, but keep your bottom in contact with your heels. Relax in this position for a count of 20, or as long as you like. Slowly roll back to a sitting position.

Just 30 minutes of exercise a day

You may find it hard to motivate yourself to exercise on a daily or regular basis, but consider this: PMS destroys the quality of your life and an exercise programme – even one as simple as 15 to 30 minutes' walking a day – can significantly ease your symptoms.

If you hate exercising or simply haven't got the time, just half an hour a day of moderate exercise is really all you need to do. And you don't even have to join a gym or buy a home workout video, unless you want to of course. Experts are now saying that half an hour of moderate, gentle exercise that can be easily incorporated into your day, such as walking in your lunch hour, doing housework, swimming or cycling or playing an active game with your kids, mowing the lawn, cleaning the windows and so on, is enough to build and maintain good health.

Half an hour a day is a small price to pay for your health and well-being; and as we've seen, that half an hour doesn't have to become a chore – you can make it a fun part of your day. So there really is no excuse now! Exercise can help you to beat PMS. Make it a part of your life.

6

Natural progesterone

For oestrogen and progesterone to work well, they need to be in balance, but increasingly today this appears to be a difficult condition to fulfil. Stress, a poor diet, lack of exercise and exposure to xenoestrogens (see Chapter 8) can all trigger higher than normal levels of oestrogen. The problems associated with oestrogen excess in women don't just include symptoms of PMS – they can affect blood sugar levels and thyroid function, and can also increase the risk of breast and endometrial cancer.

It is important to realize that oestrogen is a vital hormone for your health and well-being. It is the imbalance of oestrogen and progesterone, and not excess oestrogen, that is thought to be responsible for many PMS symptoms. However, since low levels of progesterone are also thought to be the cause of PMS in a great majority of women, some experts believe that giving supplementary progesterone is the answer. Research has shown that supplementary progesterone can ease the following symptoms: mood swings, irritability, depression, anxiety, breast tenderness, water retention, weight gain, sluggish thyroid and insomnia.

Progesterone therapy as a cure for PMS first came to public attention in the 1940s when British gynaecologist Katharina Dalton (who was also the first to define the syndrome of PMS) pioneered the use of progesterone suppositories to treat PMS. Since then, with methods and dosages adjusted, progesterone has been used as an effective treatment not just for PMS, but for a number of other hormone-related conditions – including menopausal symptoms, endometriosis and ovarian cysts.

At first progesterone was given by injection or as a suppository, but today it comes in cream, capsule or liquid form as well as a vaginal or rectal suppository. In the great majority of cases, progesterone therapy is given at the time when the body would typically manufacture its own progesterone at around day 10 to 15 of a cycle, and ending on the day before menstruation. No progesterone would be given in the first half of the cycle, from the first day of menstruation until ovulation, as during this time the body does not produce much progesterone anyway. By applying progesterone in this two-weeks on, two-weeks off pattern, it is possible to mimic the body's normal cycle of progesterone production and by so doing balance hormones.

The progesterone controversy

Although many women with PMS find relief when using progesterone therapy, the treatment remains controversial, with arguments raging for and against. These arguments centre on the fact that if extra progesterone needs to be given to eliminate PMS, then all women with PMS must be deficient in progesterone – but this is not the case. Some studies show that not all women with PMS have reduced levels of progesterone or, for that matter, too much oestrogen in relation to progesterone. And, as with much of the other research on PMS, some studies show that progesterone works while others claim that it does not.

Despite the numerous studies that have been undertaken and the strongly held views of many clinicians and patients that progesterone significantly improves PMS symptoms, there is still no convincing evidence yet to provide a strong basis for this treatment approach, nor are there any long-term studies of its safety.

Natural versus synthetic progesterone

Some of the confusion concerning progesterone therapy may lie in the fact that research on progesterone and synthetic progesterone is often grouped together, whereas the reality is that the two substances are very different.

The *synthetic version*, which is most widely prescribed, is not really progesterone at all; it is a progestin. Progestins are synthetic progesterone-like compounds manufactured by pharmaceutical companies. They can also be found in birth control pills and various forms of hormone replacement therapies with brand names such as Provera, Depo-Provera and Megace.

Natural progesterone (unlike synthetic progesterone which is manufactured in a laboratory) is made from a substance found in wild yams and soya beans that is converted into progesterone that is nearly identical to that which the body produces. Brand names include Prometrium, Pro-Gest and Crinone.

Both natural and synthetic progesterone will exert hormonal effects and oppose oestrogen dominance, but since the synthetic version is not an exact copy of your own oestrogen, it cannot provide all the benefits of natural progesterone, which include protection against breast cancer. Synthetic progesterone may also contribute some negative effects because it is far more powerful than your own natural progesterone and is metabolized as foreign substances into toxic metabolites. These synthetic progesterones can gravely interfere with your own natural progesterone, create other hormone-related health problems, and further exacerbate oestrogen dominance. Side-effects of synthetic progesterone include increased risk of cancer, abnormal menstrual flow, nausea, depression and fluid retention.

In short, taking synthetic progesterone to ease PMS is a bit like punching yourself in the stomach to relieve a cramp. In severe cases it might help, but in others it can make things far worse. On the other hand, natural progesterone, because it functions gently like real progesterone in your body, can help ease mood swings, ease breast tenderness and water retention and improve sleep. Until recently, pharmaceutical companies have been more interested in conducting research on synthetic progestins, so you may find that your doctor suggests synthetic progestins. If he or she does, you might want to discuss the use of natural progesterone as a possible alternative.

Note: The body easily converts natural progesterone into the identical molecule made by the body. Adverse side-effects are very rare. If taken inappropriately, natural progesterone might slightly alter the timing of the menstrual cycle. Always consult your doctor before using it.

Oral progesterone versus cream

Natural progesterone comes in several forms, including capsules, a topical cream that can be rubbed on your skin, vaginal suppositories, and sublingual drops that are placed under the tongue. In whatever form it comes, however, you will not be able to buy it over the counter as it is only available on prescription. Many experts recommend the topical cream rather than the capsules because the cream is easily absorbed and gradually released into the body in a

43

way that is similar to the ovaries' natural release of progesterone. It also doesn't produce nearly as many progesterone metabolites or break-down products.

If you take oral progesterone, even if it is natural, about 90 per cent ends up as break-down products, because the capsule has to pass through your intestines and liver before its contents can be sent through to the bloodstream. And all these break-down products floating in your bloodstream have an undesirable effect. Some of them will end up on progesterone receptor sites, blocking any progesterone you do produce, so you end up becoming less sensitive to progesterone and its benefits. Over time, the build-up of break-down products puts a strain on your liver and affects your brain function, causing fatigue, concentration problems and depression. Suppositories and sublingual drops are a little better but the problem with them is that they make your progesterone levels rise, and subsequently fall, very quickly and this causes a hormonal roller-coaster – unlike the gradual release of progesterone.

Topical creams do not have any of the above problems. They do not go through your intestines and liver, and because of this, much smaller doses need to be taken: 15–30 mg in contrast to the 100–400 mg of oral progesterone. The level of break-down products is much lower, so there is no toxic build-up and the delivery of progesterone is slower and more natural. When the progesterone is applied to the skin it first absorbs into the fat underneath the skin, before being gradually released into the bloodstream in amounts that mimic the normal levels of progesterone in the body.

There are many brands of progesterone cream, but be wary of any that are available over the counter – especially those that contain wild yam extract, diosgenin or dioscorea, all of which are names for the substance extracted from wild yams and converted to progesterone. Wild yam extracts are sometimes confused with natural progesterone because natural progesterone is synthesized from the chemical compound diosgenin, which is found in soya beans and wild yams. There have been suggestions, therefore, that the use of wild yam cream (which contains diosgenin) will increase progesterone levels. This is actually incorrect, as the human body does not have the enzymes capable of converting diosgenin into progesterone. Similarly, any cream sold over the counter (not obtained on prescription) claiming to contain natural progesterone is fraudulent as products containing natural progesterone can now only be obtained on prescription. It is safer and more effective to get a prescription for a natural progesterone cream from your doctor.

Applying the cream

John R. Lee, M.D., author of *What Your Doctor May Not Tell You About Premenopause* and an expert on natural progesterone, suggests using a 1.6 cream containing 450–500 mg of progesterone per ounce. The cream should be free of herbs, phytoestrogens, synthetic progesterone and mineral oil, which can block the skin's absorption of progesterone. Dr Lee suggests using 2 oz of cream in a 16- to 18-day period beginning on day 10 or day 12 and ending on day 28 of a normal menstrual cycle. Twice a day (in the morning and in the evening) rub half a teaspoon on an area of your body that is soft and hairless – for example, the insides of your upper arm, your chest, your neck, the palms of your hands or the soles of your feet. Rotate your application areas, using a different area each time. Dr Lee also suggests that you use slightly less cream (say an eighth of a teaspoon) on day 10 or 12 and increase to larger doses (no more than half a teaspoon) on day 28. If your symptoms ease after using the cream for three months, reduce the amount of progesterone cream you use to 1 oz and see if the good results continue. Adjust if necessary.

Keeping your balance

If you start using natural progesterone cream and feel worse, you may be applying too much and need to cut back. If you start to feel better, you may also want to adjust the amount you are taking. It is a delicate balancing act and you need to listen to your body's signals to make it work for you.

Neils Lauersen, M.D., co-author of *Premenstrual Syndrome and You*, and professor of obstetrics and gynaecology at New York Medical College, claims that more than 90 per cent of patients in his practice who have tried natural progesterone have found relief. 'It is the treatment of choice in my practice. Hundreds of women who were severely handicapped by PMS have been completely symptom free with (natural) progesterone,' says Dr Lauersen. He adds that in his experience, synthetic progestins actually worsen the symptoms of PMS and that many women under his care have also found that natural progesterone can relieve and prevent menstrual cramps. And it can be of value during the premenopausal period when oestrogen production often continues unabated and the body is lacking in progesterone, causing various emotional and physical symptoms, including the rapid growth of uterine fibroids.

Reading the papers of the progesterone researchers, it is easy to get the feeling that progesterone is an all-beneficent cure-all, while oestrogen causes nothing but trouble. This cannot be entirely the case, however, since oestrogen is essential for your fertility, health and well-being and every woman will respond differently to natural progesterone therapy. You could also argue that progesterone creams, even those that claim to be natural, are not natural at all but are in fact drugs. As always, it is important to keep a sense of balance and perspective when trying to find the best ways to balance your hormones.

7

Herbs for a PMS-free life

Herbs, spices and other nutritional substances are the oldest form of medicine known to humanity. While modern or 'allopathic' medicine is barely a century old, the practice of using nature as a pharmacy can be traced back through ancient civilizations. Over many centuries, experiments with plants have yielded a vast stock of natural medicines to help us heal many ailments. Many pharmaceuticals are still derived from the extracts of wild plants, such as digitalis from the purple foxglove flower.

Historically, herbal medicine has been the main form of medicine used to treat the female cycle and hormonal problems. As such, there are many herbs available to the medical herbalist to treat period pain, PMS and the menopause. Even though some doctors still do not consider herbs as viable treatments, there is enough research[16] to show that herbs can function as gentle and effective treatments for your symptoms. Instead of overpowering your body, as conventional drugs do, herbs can gently give your body what it needs to restore balance and heal itself.

Dried herbs in tablets or capsules have to be digested, and how effectively they work depends on how efficiently your body can process and absorb them. The easiest and most effective way to take herbs is in tincture form, using approximately one teaspoon three times daily in water. In the liquid form, herbs are already dissolved and can work more quickly in your body.

Herbs that work best in treating PMS aim to correct any hormonal imbalances, but as you may not be sure which hormones are out of balance, you might want to take those that have a general balancing effect first, such as chasteberry. Many herbs can be used to treat symptoms of PMS: some to ease breast pain, reduce bloating or support the liver, which detoxifies old hormones; others to boost mood and reduce stress. There isn't enough space here to include all the herbs that might prove useful for PMS, but here are some of the most well-known ones. You can also find more information on herbs for specific symptoms in Chapter 14.

Warning: If you are pregnant or hoping to be, have a pre-existing medical condition or are taking any medication, avoid any kind of herbal treatment unless you have consulted your doctor or are under the supervision of a qualified medical herbalist. Herbs can gently give your body what it needs to restore balance and heal itself. Herbs also tend to be free of unwanted side-effects, although it is important to bear in mind that there may be contraindications and just because something is called 'natural' does not mean that it is necessarily harmless.

Too much of one herb, or the wrong mixture of herbs and certain medications, can have dangerous consequences for your health, so if you would like to try herbal remedies, it is always best to visit a qualified herbalist and follow his or her instructions. It is also a good idea to consult with your doctor to make sure that the herbal remedies you want to take will not have any adverse effects and will benefit rather than harm you.

A to Z of herbs for PMS

Black cohosh (Cimifuga racemosa)

Black cohosh has oestrogen-like actions that appear to re-balance female hormones. It was originally used by Native Americans, hence the other name by which it is known: squawroot. Because it can occupy oestrogen receptor sites, it has the ability to lower high oestrogen levels and therefore reduces the effects of oestrogen dominance. In women with low oestrogen levels, black cohosh can supply a mild oestrogenic boost. As well as balancing hormones, it also has a calming effect on the nervous system and can be helpful with PMS anxiety, stress and depression. It is also a mild painkiller and is useful for PMS headaches.

Warning: It is better to avoid this herb if you get heavy periods.

Chamomile (Matricaria chamomile)

Chamomile tea is well known for its relaxing qualities, but the herb also has natural anti-inflammatory, anti-bacterial and anti-fungal ingredients. Chamomile has been used for centuries to treat insomnia, aches and pains and anxiety. If you are not allergic to members of the aster or daisy family, try a cup of chamomile tea (made from one tablespoon of chamomile flower steeped in boiling water) three times a day, or drink ten to twenty drops of extract mixed with water two to three times a day.

Chasteberry tree (Vitex agnus castus)

Chasteberry tree extract helps to balance your hormones by working on the pituitary gland. It reduces follicle stimulating hormone and increases luteinizing hormone, which helps to balance the ratio of oestrogen to progesterone in the second half of your cycle. It can also reduce your production of prolactin. Because prolactin and progesterone tend to balance one another, reducing prolactin boosts your progesterone and this can ease PMS. Three large-scale studies[17] on a total of 4,500 women on the effect of chasteberry extract on PMS showed that at a daily dosage of 40 drops of liquid extract (35 mg of plant extract), nearly one-third of the women found relief and more than half saw marked improvement.

Warning: If you are taking the pill avoid chasteberry as its effect on prolactin could end up decreasing the pill's effectiveness.

Dandelion (Taraxacum officinale)

Loaded with beta-carotene, Vitamin C, iron, calcium, potassium and other minerals, the dandelion is an excellent diuretic that helps your body shed the excess water that contributes to PMS bloating. Dandelion also helps to stabilize blood sugar levels and stimulates and supports liver function, which is important for the breakdown of toxins and old hormones. Constipation, headaches and acne can be eased with this herb. Almost the whole plant – flowers, leaves and root – can be used for herbal treatments. Juice can be extracted from the plant, the leaves can be eaten, and tea can be made from the roots or leaves. Tinctures and extracts are also available from health food shops. You can eat the dandelions that grow in your yard or garden as long as you haven't used a pesticide (or weedkiller) on it. You will also probably want to avoid eating the leaves if you have used a synthetic lawn fertilizer. But if your yard is organic, dig in!

Dong quai (Angelica sinensis)

This Chinese herb, known as the female ginseng, has a long history. It can be helpful in treating PMS because studies[18] show that it promotes hormonal balance and can regulate sugar levels, which, as we have seen, is vital for PMS. It appears to have phytoestrogen effects, which are helpful when the problem is too much or too little oestrogen. And because dong quai also has muscle-relaxing qual-ities, it is particularly suggested for women who get premenstrual pains and cramps. You should not take this herb during menstruation or when pregnant.

Evening primrose oil

Modern herbal science has found that evening primrose oil can help correct low levels of essential fatty acids, which – as we saw in Chapter 3 – can trigger symptoms of PMS. Evening primrose oil is particularly rich in gamma linolenic acid (omega 6). Older studies[19] showed that supplementing your diet with evening primrose oil that contains GLA (gamma linolenic acid) could reduce breast discomfort. More recent studies, however, do not show this correlation. The only way to find out if evening primrose oil can help you is by trial and error.

False unicorn root

This herb is known to help restore hormonal balance and function. It exerts a mild oestrogen-like effect, boosting low levels or lowering high ones. False unicorn root is also believed to ease headaches and treat delayed periods.

Garcinia cambognia

This small tropical fruit contains HCA (hydroxy-citric acid) which encourages your body to use carbohydrates for energy rather than lay them down as fat. HCA also seems to curb appetite and may increase the rate at which you burn fat, so it may help get PMS food cravings under control. The theory is that it activates an enzyme called carnitine acetyl-transferase, which speeds up the fat-burning process.

Milk thistle (Silybum marianum)

If you have PMS, support for the liver is important since this detoxifying organ plays a big part in the breakdown and excretion of unwanted oestrogen. The liver also detoxifies harmful substances such as alcohol, nicotine and other toxins. A number of studies have shown that milk thistle helps to boost liver function and produce new liver cells as a result of the action of a flavonoid it contains called silymarin. As well as being a powerful antioxidant, milk thistle also contains linolenic acid, an essential acid that is important for relieving symptoms of PMS.

Motherwort (Lenourus cardiaca)

In the seventeenth century motherwort was highly regarded as a tonic for menstrual and labour pains. Motherwort is recommended by herbalists today as a remedy for delayed menstruation, water retention, nervous tension, and to generally ease symptoms of PMS. Motherwort can cause the uterus to contract, so should never be used during pregnancy.

Nettle

Herbalists consider the nettle a great all-round tonic for women with PMS, especially for its diuretic properties and its high nutrient content. You can take nettles as a tincture, juice or tea, but you can also eat freshly cooked nettle greens (nettles are available at some health food shops).

Siberian ginseng (Eleutherococcus senticosus)

This herb may be helpful for women with PMS because of its stress-relieving properties. It is classed as an adaptogen because it can adapt to your body's needs, helping to combat stress when you are under pressure. It also helps to support adrenal gland function and may be extremely useful when you are under physical and emotional stress.

Skullcap (Scuterlleria lateriflora)

This herb soothes the nervous system and may be especially helpful for anxiety caused by PMS, depression, irritability, headaches and insomnia. It also has anti-spasmodic qualities, which can aid liver function and ease painful periods.

St John's Wort (Hypericum perforatum)

This has been used as a medicinal herb since Greek and Roman times, but only recently has it been rediscovered as a mood enhancer for those suffering from anxiety, depression and PMS-related symptoms. Researchers believe that St John's Wort can work as an antidepressant, but without the side-effects of some of the pharmaceutical drugs. It helps make the 'feel-good' chemicals – such as serotonin – more available to the body. Although some women say they feel better in a matter of days, in general it takes about two to three months before the full benefits can be experienced. Do not drink alcohol or take any antidepressant drugs or the contraceptive pill if you use this herb.

Valerian

Valerian is believed to have a calming effect and is often recommended to relieve anxiety and depression caused by stress or nervous tension – hence its use in treating PMS. It can ease cramps and muscle pain and is helpful for tension headaches. Valerian is well known as a sleep aid, with studies showing that it can increase sleep quality because it shortens the amount of time it takes to fall asleep.

8
Your PMS detox boost

Your PMS detox boost isn't about speedy weight loss or fasting, but about trying to avoid unnecessary toxins, chemicals and pollutants that can clog up your system, unsettle your hormones and make your PMS worse.

Man-made toxins

It is estimated that since the 1950s over 3,500 new man-made chemicals have found their way into the food we regularly eat. This puts a huge burden on the liver, kidneys, adrenals and skin; some of the major man-made culprits are listed below:

- Chemicals and additives in food.
- Over-the-counter drugs.
- Heavy metals such as lead, cadmium and aluminium used in industrial processes, petrol, cooking utensils, domestic water pipes, dental fillings, cigarette smoke, old paintwork and antacid medication.
- Pollutants from carpets, cleaning materials, insecticides, fumes from gas boilers, insulation materials, paints, washing machines, car exhausts, electromagnetic fields (EMF) from TVs, mobile phones, microwave ovens, fridges, electric clocks.
- EDCs or xenoestrogens.

Your body does not need or want these chemicals and toxins and has to work very hard to metabolize and get rid of them, and in the process you lose vital nutrients – nutrients you need to beat PMS.

Xenoestrogens

Xenoestrogens or endocrine (hormone)-disturbing chemicals (EDCs) are petrochemicals from pesticides or plastics that are widely recognized as highly toxic even in the smallest doses. They are particularly bad if you have PMS because they are classified as hormone disruptors, with a molecular structure that is similar to oestrogen. This gives them the ability to function in the same way as oestrogen in the body.

As soon as xenoestrogens enter your body either through your mouth or nose or skin, EDCs interfere with your hormones and prevent them from doing their job correctly in various ways. EDCs attach themselves to oestrogen receptor sites and encourage the creation of brand-new oestrogen and hamper the liver's ability to dismantle and excrete old hormones, increasing the oestrogen build-up.

Just how damaging the effect of these fake hormones can be on your body becomes clear when you see how they can affect wildlife. Research has shown that male birds exposed to EDCs become sterile. In some cases they even switch gender, and female animals may lose their fertility. Many experts believe that the increasing occurrence of progesterone deficiency and infertility could be a direct result of exposure to EDCs. The hormonal imbalance they can trigger may be responsible not just for PMS, but for loss of libido, mood swings and an increased risk of cancer.

How to avoid the worst toxins and other risk factors

If you are suffering from oestrogen excess, the last thing you need is to get more oestrogen from your environment. And even if you are deficient in oestrogen, you still don't want these toxins clogging up receptor sites and blocking the entry of good natural oestrogen.

There are countless detox programmes and diets recommended to cleanse your system, but they aren't usually a good idea as they slow your metabolism and are hard to stick to. You don't really need to go on fasts, retreats or harsh regimes or take supplements to protect yourself from toxicity. The best way to protect against xenoestrogens is to keep your body's own self-purifying system in good order by giving your liver, kidneys and adrenals (the key organs of detoxification in your body) nutritional support from a healthy diet, and combining this with regular exercise to encourage the flushing out of toxins. You should also eliminate or cut back on your exposure to the following sources of toxins.

Saturated fat

The fat you get from meats, poultry, eggs and dairy products is more likely to contain high amounts of xenoestrogens due to the hormones, antibiotics and pesticides that are used to grow, feed or produce them. Your best bet is to cut back or eliminate your intake of red meat while eating limited amounts of non-fat dairy products and hormone-free poultry. Fish that come from fish farms are safest. You should also avoid trans-fatty acids found in many commercial foods such as pastries, pies, chips and cakes as these have been directly linked to an increased risk of obesity and heart disease.

Petroleum

It is impossible to avoid exposure to the chemicals in petroleum completely, but you can achieve a certain amount of damage control. On days when pollution is high, close the windows in your home and use an air conditioner as a filter. Stay away from traffic as much as possible and limit your contact with major sources of pollution such as factories. Also minimize your exposure to solvents, glues, adhesives or soaps made from petrochemical-based emulsifiers as well as air fresheners, fabric softeners and perfumed soaps.

Plastics

Avoid as far as is possible food and drinks in plastic containers or wrapped in plastic. Plastics are a major petrochemical by-product, and the less exposure you have to it the better. Don't store any fatty foods (cheese, meat, etc.) in plastic wrap or clingfilm. Because xenoestrogens are lipophilic (fat loving) they will tend to absorb into food with a high fat content. Remove food from plastic wrapping as soon as possible and don't heat food in plastic, especially in a microwave, since some kinds of plastics will release xenoestrogens into the food or beverage when heated; use ceramic dishes or cups instead. Also, wear natural fibres instead of plastic-based polyester or vinyl.

Additives and preservatives

Along with alcohol and caffeine, your body sees sugar, salt, food colourings, preservatives and additives as unwanted toxins that increase your risk of hypertension, heart disease, diabetes and cancer. Avoid these as much as possible. Processed ready-cooked, canned and refined foods are often high in these substances, and high in additives, so limit the amount you consume. Additives in food have been linked to a variety of health problems, including head-aches and allergies. Highly refined foods tend to have substances added to enhance flavour and prolong life, and these additives are known to be harmful to health and upset hormonal balance. The additives that cause the most damage are monosodium glutamate

(MSG), artificial colourings, sorbate, sulphates, aspartame, butylated hydroxyanisole and butylated hydroxytoluene. Get into the habit of reading food labels to check what you are actually taking into your body. Watch out for alternative names. For instance, sodium is another name for salt, animal fat is saturated fat, and sugar has many pseudonyms: sucrose, fructose, dextrose or maple syrup to name but a few. As a rule of thumb, if you cannot understand a label, cannot see any natural ingredients, or the list of chemical ingredients is so long there's barely enough room for it, leave it on the shelf.

Non-organic fruits and vegetables

As far as possible, buy organic fruit and vegetables that are naturally grown and have not been chemically treated. There are thousands of types of insecticide, herbicide and fungicide approved for use in the UK and USA, and some fruits and vegetables are sprayed as many as ten times.

Tap water

The World Health Organization (WHO) has claimed that 80 per cent of the world's illness would be eliminated if we drank pure water. WHO estimates that 80 per cent of this illness is caused by contaminated drinking water. It is claimed that as many as 60,000 different chemicals, metals and toxins now contaminate our water supply. Ideally, you should purify drinking water in the home with a water filter jug, readily available from department stores and health food shops. Alternatively, buy water bottled in glass. (Avoid plastic because plastic compounds are leached from the bottle into the water. There is also an increasing environmental concern about the transport and disposal of plastic water bottles, which could contribute significantly to landfill.) Or drink cooled boiled tap water to get rid of the bacteria and limescale. If you are still drinking tap water and suspect you have got lead pipes, use only the cold for drinking and cooking.

Overcooked food

Avoid overcooking your food as it can destroy vital nutrients – nutrients you need to fight toxins. Try grilling instead of frying, lightly steam vegetables instead of boiling them, and avoid all aluminium cookware.

Smoking

Cigarette smoking is the biggest cause of preventable disease. Studies show that passive smoking has its risks too. According to research published in the *Journal of the American Medical Association* (January 1998), just 30 minutes in the company of smokers can damage your heart by reducing its ability to pump blood. Smoking is an anti-nutrient and has high levels of chemicals, such as cadmium – a heavy toxic metal that can stop the utilization of zinc needed for a healthy menstrual cycle. It is well known that smoking is linked to menstrual irregularities, early menopause, heart disease, cancer and poor health in general, and if you are concerned about your PMS and you are a smoker, you should consider why you are taking into your body something that is only going to make things worse.

To protect your health in the future, nothing is as effective as stopping smoking completely. There are many books about quitting smoking, but arguably the most successful method is to go cold turkey. Make the decision to smoke your last cigarette. The nicotine will pass out of your system in a matter of days and the challenge then will be to find healthy habits to replace smoking. A healthy diet and regular exercise and some pampering can all help you stay strong. Chewing some sugar-free gum or drinking some water or jumping on the spot are all techniques that ex-smokers have used to beat the cravings. If you need something to do with your hands, why not buy some worry beads!

Chlorine

Chlorine and chlorinated compounds are potent xenoestrogens, and bleach, cleansers and certain deodorants are the main source of chlorine in our environment. Buy natural cleaning products to reduce the number of potentially xenoestrogenic chemicals in your home. Or use the tried and tested methods your granny used when there were far less chemicals around, such as white vinegar and lemon for stain removal, washing soda instead of commercial soda, or chemical-free liquid soaps and detergents.

Aldehydes

Use natural toiletries, make-up, nail polish, deodorants and creams whenever you can. Scientists are investigating a link between the chemicals in deodorants and antiperspirants and breast cancer. The answer is to buy chemical free where you can.

Tampons

Tampons, especially super-absorbent brands, may dry out the vagina, making the transfer of toxins into the bloodstream easier. It is best to use towels instead, but if you need to use tampons, try to manage with the lowest possible absorbency and make sure that you change them regularly – say every four to six hours. Some studies of different kinds of tampons have found that the only ones that did not produce toxins were those made of 100 per cent cotton, so if possible use these.

Nonylphenols

These are by-products of surfactants found in detergents, cosmetics, pesticides and herbicides. They can also be found in nonoxynol 9, a common spermicide found in diaphragm jellies and condoms. To avoid nonylphenols, get rid of lawn sprays, bug sprays, flea removal products and all other pesticides and herbicides. Buy organic pesticide-free produce, use environmentally safe detergents and avoid spermicides.

Electromagnetic exposure

Commonplace items in your bedroom – from alarm clocks, televisions and videos to power sockets near your bed – may help increase the potential of electromagnetic exposure. Purchase battery-operated clocks and radios or unplug electrical sockets in the evening. If your work involves VDUs, make sure you take regular breaks – get up and walk around – every 30 minutes or so. It is also a good idea to go for a walk in a park or a green place at least once a day. Trees give out energizing oxygen. Surround your home and workplace with plants if you live in a city or busy town. NASA research has shown that the following plants can extract fumes, chemicals and smoke from the air: peace lilies, dwarf banana plants, spider plants, weeping fig, geraniums and chrysanthemums.

Stress

Symptoms usually flare up when you are under stress. If you are having a bad week at work, are not sleeping properly, or have to make major decisions, signs of toxicity can worsen. This is because stress causes your energy reserves to be channelled away from your body's detoxification mechanisms. The stress management techniques in Chapter 10 should help.

Synthetic oestrogens

If you are trying to avoid xenoestrogens, the last thing you should be doing is taking one synthetic oestrogen into your body via oestrogen replacement or the birth control pill. Man-made oestrogen can have negative effects on your body, so if your doctor tells you that you are oestrogen-deficient, opt for a form of natural oestrogen replacement. As for birth control, you might want to consider a non-chemical method if you can.

Weight gain

While we don't yet know enough about EDCs, we do know that for some reason they love fat. They are stored in body fat, and overweight people tend to have higher concentrations. Weight gain not only increases your body's toxic load, it also triggers or makes worse PMS symptoms. In fact, weight management can be such an important part of beating PMS that the next chapter is devoted to it.

9

Easing symptoms with weight loss

Many women gain weight during their menstrual cycle and/or during PMS. This weight gain may be caused by consuming excess calories as a result of food cravings or by water retention. Unfortunately, the more overweight you are, the more likely you are to suffer from PMS. This is because excess weight can lead to higher insulin levels as well as higher levels of other hormones, which can trigger hormonal imbalance and symptoms of PMS. Research[20] has shown a clear link between excess weight, hormonal imbalance and symptoms of PMS. It is a vicious circle. Not only can PMS trigger weight gain, but weight gain increases the likelihood of symptoms. The solution is to keep an eye on your weight.

Both slim and overweight women can and do suffer from PMS, but if you have weight to lose (see BMI chart on p. 62 to determine if you do), weight loss is recommended. This isn't easy, but you may find that you lose weight naturally if you are following the healthy eating and exercise guidelines given previously, which help balance your blood sugar levels, reduce food cravings and speed up your metabolism. If, however, you are eating a nutritious diet and exercising regularly, but still can't seem to lose weight after three or four months, the following natural weight-loss tips are designed to help you shed the pounds.

Tips for losing weight

Write things down

Keeping a food diary can focus you. It makes you think about whether your diet is triggering your symptoms or making them worse. A food diary also gives you a feeling of control. However, the most important thing about writing down what you eat is the awareness it brings, and the way it encourages you to notice what you are doing. You cannot change habits of which you are not aware.

Adjust your appetite

Eating more than you need is one of the most common causes of weight gain, so if your eyes are bigger than your stomach, try the following techniques:

- Take time over your meals. Put your knife and fork down after each mouthful and chew food slowly.
- If you think you need to eat more, wait 10 or 15 minutes to see if you are still hungry. It takes quite a while for your brain to recognize when your stomach is full.
- Never shop or cook when you are hungry. Keep a supply of healthy, low-fat, low-sugar snacks near by, such as apples and nuts, dried fruit and low-fat yogurt, so you never get really hungry.
- Around six meals a day is best for losing weight and for keeping hunger at bay. If there is a long gap between meals, blood sugar levels fall too low, leaving you feeling tired, craving sugar and lacking in energy and concentration. Give your body food every few hours to boost your metabolic rate and keep blood sugar levels stable.
- Stop eating several hours before you go to bed, say 8 p.m. A light snack, say a cracker and a glass of skimmed milk, if you feel peckish is OK, but not a heavy meal. This is because your body needs to rest, not digest, when you sleep. It does not make sense to eat a great deal of food when all you are going to do is sleep. The earlier in the day you eat, the more likely you are to burn off calories, even if you aren't active.
- Make nutrient-rich foods such as wholegrains, fruit and vegetables the staples of your diet. They are filling and satisfying, but low in calories.

Beat food cravings

Many women with PMS find that they have strong sugar and carbohydrate cravings a week or so before their period, and this plays havoc with their weight-loss plans. High-calorie sugary carbohydrates, such as cakes, chocolate, crisps, sweets and pastries, are the foods we often crave because they send blood sugar levels rocketing, so giving an instant energy boost.

However, the boost is short-lived as it leads to an overproduction of insulin followed by a dip in blood sugar, leaving you tired and sleepy and craving the foods all over again. If you suffer from food cravings, all the appetite control tips listed above will help keep cravings at bay. You can also really help yourself by eating little and often, and by using the glycaemic index (GI) when making your carbohydrate food choices. If you want to eat a food with a high GI, make sure you balance it with some protein and fat to slow down the release of sugar. (See also the food cravings entry in Chapter 14: A to Z of common symptoms and natural ways to treat them.)

Do I have weight to lose?

Right now, the best tool for deciding if your current weight is healthy is the BMI – body mass index. Essentially, the BMI is a formula that relates to body fat, and is better at predicting the risk of disease than body weight alone. If you want to know your BMI, multiply your weight in pounds by 700 and divide the product by your height in inches squared:

BMI = weight x 700 divided by height x height

For example, if you weigh 200 pounds and your height is 5 ft 7 in, your BMI would be 31 (200 x 700 divided by 67 x 67 or 14000 divided by 4489). If the result of your number is between 19 and 25, you are at a healthy weight and your goal should be to maintain this weight. A number of 27 or higher is an indication that you are overweight. A BMI of lower than 19 suggests you are underweight.

The BMI can also be used to help you determine your weight loss goal. If your BMI is over 25, calculate the weight at which you would need to be to have a BMI of 25 (25 x your height x your height divided by 700). Then subtract your answer from your current weight to find your weight loss goal. Is this weight loss realistic? Much depends on your age and your circumstances, and you may have to decide on a long-term goal, something to be accomplished over the next few years rather than the next few months. Whatever your goal weight, the loss of one or two pounds a week is a realistic and healthy expectation and sets you on the path to finding your natural weight.

A good night's sleep

Sleep is important as lack of sleep disrupts your hormones, triggering changes in metabolism so that you end up not processing food as well as you could. It is thought that lack of sleep is linked with higher levels of cortisol, which can throw the metabolism out of balance. Other studies have shown lack of sleep can have a negative effect on carbohydrate metabolism and endocrine function, lowering glucose tolerance and making it more difficult to convert carbohydrates into energy. This makes it more likely that fats and sugars are stored as unwanted extra pounds. Further studies have established a link between lack of sleep and increased appetite, largely because cortisol is important in appetite control. (See Chapter 10 for tips on getting a good night's sleep.)

Green tea

Drinking four cups of green tea each day is also said to help you lose weight. Studies at the American Society for Clinical Nutrition found that one of the compounds in green tea, catechol, increases metabolism and reduces the amount of fat your body absorbs by as much as 30 per cent. Green tea is rich in natural antioxidants which fight the damaging effects of free radicals. Green tea also contains Vitamin B5, which plays a key role in the body's metabolism, and Vitamins B1 and B2 which are essential for releasing energy from food.

Water

Drinking a glass of water before you eat can also aid weight loss because you feel fuller. Water helps to flush out toxins and waste, but it is also very important for weight loss. Fat can be broken down only in the presence of water, and water can also have a direct impact on energy. We may reach for a sugar fix when what we really need to do is rehydrate the body.

Soup

Having a bowl of soup may also help you lose weight. American researchers at Johns Hopkins University in Baltimore found that people who chose soup as a starter consumed 25 per cent less fat in the following main course than those who chose a high-fat starter.

Weight loss supplements

In the majority of cases you can get all the nutrients you need for weight loss from your healthy diet and a multivitamin and mineral supplement, but deficiency in the following nutrients has been linked with an increased risk of weight gain:

- B vitamins are important for weight loss because they are involved in energy production, helping to control fat metabolism and digestion. It is best to get your B vitamins from your diet (foods such as wholegrains, nuts, fish, vegetables and low-fat dairy foods are rich in B vitamins), but if you think you may be deficient, the best way to make sure you are getting enough Vitamin B is a good B complex supplement.
- Chromium is needed for the metabolism of sugar. Without chromium, insulin is less effective in controlling blood sugar levels, which means it is harder to burn off food as fuel and more is stored as fat. Chromium may also help to control levels of fat and cholesterol in the blood, according to one study. Good food sources of chromium include wholegrains, bananas, carrots, cabbage, mushrooms and strawberries.
- Manganese helps with the absorption of fats and also works to stabilize blood sugar levels. It also functions in many enzymes, including those involved in burning energy. Foods rich in manganese include green leafy vegetables, pecans, pulses and wholegrains.
- Magnesium aids in the production of insulin and helps to regulate blood sugar levels, so it is important that this mineral is in good supply. Foods rich in magnesium include green leafy vegetables, nuts and seeds and soya beans.
- Zinc is important because it can help to control appetite, and a deficiency can cause a loss of taste and smell. Make sure that your multivitamin and mineral supplement contains zinc, and include more zinc-rich foods in your diet – such as green leafy vegetables, nuts, seeds, wholegrains and eggs.
- Other nutritional supplements often recommended to help you lose weight include potassium, calcium, and co-enzyme Q10, all of which are important in the production of energy; EFAs (essential fatty acids) for appetite control; psyllium husks for fibre to promote a feeling of being full; kelp, which contains minerals that can help with weight loss; lecithin capsules that can help

break down fat; spirulina that can help to stabilize blood sugar; Vitamin C to speed up a slow metabolism; boron to speed up the burning of calories (raisins and onions are good sources); cinnamon to balance blood sugars; and the amino acids L-ornithine, L-arginine and L-lysine, as research has shown that weight loss can be improved with a combination of these.

If you want to take any additional supplements to boost efforts at weight loss, you should consult your doctor or a nutritionist. You also need to remember that these supplements will not help you a great deal unless you combine them with a healthy diet and regular exercise.

Slow and gradual weight loss is the key

Eating a healthy diet and exercising regularly is the most successful way to lose weight and beat your symptoms, but it takes time – typically a good three to six months – before you start to see the benefits.

Three to six months may seem a long time if you want to lose weight, but there isn't a quick fix to weight loss. You need to edge slowly and steadily towards your weight loss goal and aim for a weight loss of no more than one or two pounds a week, as this has been shown to be the most effective way to lose weight. If weight loss isn't fast, it can be tempting to diet, but diets rarely work in the long term as they slow your metabolism right down because your body thinks there is a shortage of food. Steer clear of diets and focus your energy on eating more healthy nutritious foods. The only way to lose weight safely and keep it off in the long term is to lose it slowly and gradually by changing your eating habits and exercising regularly, and ensuring that these new healthier habits become a way of life.

You may find that around three months is also the amount of time it takes for you to see a real improvement in your symptoms. Although you may feel better in a few weeks, typically it will take at least two menstrual cycles to really feel the benefits, as this is the optimum amount of time for dietary changes to take effect and exercise routines and nutritional supplements and herbs to work their magic. This makes sense if you think about it, as your body and mind need time to adjust to new habits.

According to nutritionists and psychologists, it typically takes around three months to replace unhealthy dietary and lifestyle habits with healthier ones. So try not to get despondent if you still get symptoms during the first, or even the second, month after making changes to your diet and lifestyle. Remind yourself that your body and mind are still adjusting and that old habits die hard. If you want to feel better, you need to stick with it.

10

The PMS/stress connection

Stress can trigger symptoms of PMS or make them worse.[21] This is because when you are stressed your body manufactures stress hormones to help you respond to the stress, but these are manufactured at the expense of your progesterone supply. In other words, stress eats up your progesterone supply and helps to plunge you into oestrogen dominance, which, as we have seen, can trigger symptoms of PMS.

It is interesting to note that when women with PMS are premenstrual, they are known to see daily stressors as more stressful than women without PMS do. What is more, it seems that women with PMS tend to experience more stress than women without PMS. As with weight gain in the previous chapter, it seems that once again we have a vicious circle; not only does PMS predispose a woman to stress, but stress can trigger PMS.

Stress and your adrenals

The adrenal glands, two organs that sit just on top of the kidneys, play an important part in the stress response. When you feel stressed they are responsible for releasing special stress hormones – adrenaline and cortisol – into your bloodstream. Cortisol helps to release energy, and in times of stress it is released at about 20 times its normal rate, but there is a problem with this. Cortisol is made from progesterone, and if you are chronically stressed this can trigger oestrogen dominance. Cortisol also slows down the thyroid gland, which can lead to weight gain, fatigue, low sex drive, headaches and other PMS symptoms.

Stress hormones are essential to our survival as they can give us the energy to fight or escape, but the trouble with typical modern stressors is that they often don't require a physical response. Sadly, in most cases, such as a difficult situation at work or sitting in a traffic jam, all you can do is sit there while your stress hormones run riot. This is fine now and again, but if you are exposed to high levels of stress hormones day in day out, this can have a damaging effect on your heart, your stomach, your psychological health and your hormonal balance. Your adrenal glands will also become exhausted and eventually give up, and you may find yourself suffering from fatigue, aches and pains, sugar cravings and a weakened immune system. Bear in mind that if you are low in progesterone, you can have the same experience because if progesterone levels are low this results in a poor supply of stress hormones, which makes you also feel tired and susceptible to disease.

In the long term, it is vital for your health and well-being that you keep your adrenal glands healthy and do not over-use your stress hormones. The first thing in boosting the health of your adrenals is to eat a healthy diet to give your body the tools it needs to perform optimally. Diet is the foundation of good health and it cannot be overestimated in relation to stress.

Certain nutrients, such as zinc, the B vitamins – especially B5 and B6 – Vitamin C and the essential fatty acids can be extremely helpful if stress is a problem and they will help to boost the functioning of your adrenal glands. You should be getting these nutrients from your healthy PMS diet and your multivitamin and mineral supplement, but if you are under stress you might want to add in B vitamins, essential fats and plenty of Vitamin C as when you are stressed you lose more Vitamin C than at any other time. Vitamin C is vital for keeping your immune system strong.

In order to keep your adrenals from burning out you also need to be able to distinguish between what is a real stress or emergency and what isn't. Many of the things we get worked up about are not really that important, so it might also help to have a rethink about what drives you mad. Changing your attitude and identifying stress triggers can be extremely helpful, but if you still find it hard to cope with stress it is important to find ways to relieve it before it makes PMS worse. Regular exercise is a great stress-buster. Studies show it can reduce the impact of stress, relax the body and boost mood. Deep breathing exercises, meditation, yoga and tai-chi are other ways to calm your body and mind.

The following are some tried and tested stress-busting techniques you might want to use when you feel overwhelmed – but playing a musical instrument, dancing, writing in your diary, watching a funny DVD or anything that specifically helps you to relax and unwind are also highly recommended.

Instant stress-busters you can use any time, anywhere

Take a deep breath

Close your eyes and take a deep breath. Visualize yourself being in peaceful, tranquil surroundings such as the beach.

Concentrate on your breathing and slow it down to a 10-second cycle, 6 breaths a minute. Inhale for five seconds, then exhale for five seconds. Do this for about two to five minutes.

Focus on something peaceful and soothing in your environment. You may choose a flower, a colour or anything that soothes you.

If this doesn't work, jog on the spot, punch something like a cushion or count to 10.

Talk to friends, family or partners

If you don't feel you can talk to anyone you know, a trained counsellor may help you get in touch with your feelings and give you tips on how to deal with stress.

Fill out your personal space

Shrinking away from other people creates tension, so consciously relax your body: start with the shoulders and let yourself settle into your feet or your seat as if there were no one else around. Close your eyes or keep them slightly unfocused and turned downwards. Now imagine that you are expanding into the space just surrounding your body, flowing into it with every exhaling breath, taking more space for yourself.

Try herbal remedies

Valerian is helpful for stress-related anxiety and insomnia. It has been shown to help people fall asleep faster, sleep better and longer without causing loss of concentration.

Or drink some kombucha tea, which contains stress-busting B vitamins and other micronutrients and is made from a bacteria yeast culture.

One of the best herbs for relieving tension is chamomile as it has a gentle sedative effect. Drink a cup any time that you feel tense to help you relax. If you drink a cup before you go to bed, this can help you to sleep.

Take time out

For five minutes every hour, try to 'shut down' and think of nothing but your perfect situation. This could be a dream holiday, ideal partner, or simply thinking about doing nothing at all. You will be surprised at how effectively this can lower stress levels. Daydreaming is a natural stress-busting technique. Allow your mind to wander for five minutes if you feel tense – maybe using your favourite picture or happy memory to help you drift off.

Ayurvedic techniques

Try this Ayurvedic technique for soothing the brain: for as long as possible, gently massage the point above your nose in the middle of the forehead in a very light circular movement.

Aromatherapy

Certain aromas are thought to activate the production of the brain's 'feel-good' chemical serotonin. Put a few drops of the following aromatherapy oils on a tissue to sniff when you feel stress levels rising: jasmine, neroli, lavender, chamomile, ylang ylang, vetiver, clary sage. You may also want to use essential oils in your bath to help you unwind. When you feel tense, try one of the following: three drops of patchouli oil and three drops of sandalwood, three drops of rosewood and three drops of clary sage, or two drops of vetiver and jasmine. Or you might like to try putting two drops of peppermint or lemon essential oil on to a tissue and inhaling it when you feel stressed. If you prefer, you could also burn these oils in a vaporizer to help clarify and invigorate the room.

De-clutter

Mess creates confusion and a sense of loss of power. If your desk/home/car is messy and disorganized, have a good clear-out and tidy-up. You'll instantly feel more in control.

Break old habits

Many stresses are habitual. If you start to feel anxious or stressed out, do something out of character. Stop what you are doing and do something else. Or take a minute to take stock and work out why you are feeling uptight.

70

Release the tension

Do you hunch your shoulders when you are stressed? Do you tighten your fists? Do you cross your arms? Do you wrap one leg around the other? Become aware of the way that your body reacts when you are under stress. Then, when you feel yourself going into that stress position, do the opposite – release your shoulders, stretch out your hands, uncross your arms or legs, and don't forget to breathe. Stop frowning: relax your jaw by gently resting the tip of your tongue for a second behind your top front teeth. At the same time, try to consciously relax the facial muscles and let the shoulders drop down and away from your ears by an inch or two – you will be amazed to find how you were holding that tension in your body.

Stroke your pet

If you have a pet, stroke it. It has been proven to lower blood pressure and stress levels. If you haven't got a pet, why not give someone you love a hug – it will have the same effect.

Write it down

When it all seems too much, grab a pen and paper and write down what you need to do. Listing things on paper will also help focus your mind, helping you think clearly about what is a priority, what can wait, and what can be delegated to someone else. Once a job has been dealt with, be sure to cross it off the list. It is satisfying and stress-busting to watch your list shrink!

Get a good night's sleep

One of the simplest and easiest ways to de-stress is to get a good night's sleep.

Lack of sleep doesn't just make it harder for you to cope with life's stressors, it can also make PMS worse because it increases the blood sugar problems that are known to trigger the condition. Sleep and stress are linked. The less sleep you get, the more stressed you feel and the more likely you are to experience symptoms. To make things even more difficult, during the PMS phase of your cycle you are less likely to get a good night's sleep because your melatonin/serotonin levels drop just before ovulation.[22] Melatonin and serotonin are neurotransmitters that govern your sleep cycle, and if you have PMS, the chances are that you are lacking in melatonin and serotonin, setting the stage for insomnia, night waking and poor-quality sleep.

If you are not sleeping properly you may find yourself moody and suffering from headaches, fatigue and lack of concentration – which sounds very much like PMS, doesn't it? The answer is to make sure you get good-quality sleep every night by following the tips below:

Boost your serotonin levels

If your serotonin levels are high you will feel happy and calm in the day, and when night comes the serotonin will convert to melatonin and you will sleep soundly. If you have got PMS, the chances are that you are low in serotonin/melatonin. Fortunately, you can eat foods that boost your serotonin. Serotonin is manufactured within your body from the amino acid tryptophan and this is found in many foods, notably eggs, cheese, milk, lean meat, fish, soya beans and potatoes. That is why the old advice to drink a glass of low-fat or skimmed warm milk before you sleep can work wonders. You might also want to consider adding a couple of crackers or a slice of bread to your bedtime snack to help you sleep well. This is because complex carbohydrates, such as rice, oats and wheat, encourage insulin to be released, and when insulin is released, tryptophan is too.

In order for tryptophan to convert to serotonin it needs Vitamin B6, so you need to ensure that you have enough Vitamin B6 in your diet. You can get B6 from foods such as spinach, fish, lentils, avocados, carrots and potatoes. Increase your Vitamin B6 supplements in the premenstrual period, especially if you find that you feel depressed at this time.

Any food that is rich in minerals, especially calcium, magnesium and silicon, induces a calming action on the mind but a deficiency can lead to sleep problems. Try to include more such foods in your diet. Foods rich in these minerals include watercress, broccoli, parsley, leeks, spinach, almonds, sesame seeds, sunflower seeds, dried figs, pulses, beans, lentils, brown rice, peaches, bananas, dates, avocados, raisins and sea vegetables.

Get plenty of exposure to light

Light is necessary for serotonin production. Make sure you go out in the daylight each day or consider buying a light box (see Chapter 12).

Cultivate good sleeping habits

Whether you struggle with falling asleep, or wake in the middle of the night (most typical for women with PMS), some basic good-sleep strategies will help you sleep better. These include:

- Sticking to a regular sleep–wake pattern, even at weekends. Ideally you should aim to be in bed around 11 p.m. as studies show that people who sleep before midnight tend to wake more refreshed than those who go to bed in the small hours.
- Deciding how much sleep you need. Eight hours is enough for most people, but you may need more or less than this to feel alert and refreshed. If you want to nap during the day, research shows that 25 minutes is the optimum time for a nap. Research also shows that between six and eight hours is the optimum amount of sleep needed for most adults.
- Making sure your mattress and bed are comfortable. Use your bed only for sleeping and sex, so that you associate it with rest and pleasure when you get into bed. Block out noise and light, as light will impair the production of melatonin. Sleep in a well-ventilated cool but not cold room (around 55–65 degrees) as body temperature naturally falls at night, to promote feelings of sleepiness.
- Winding down for an hour or so before you go to bed. Activity delays melatonin production. Try taking a warm bath, doing yoga, having a quiet chat, making love, doing relaxation exercises, or drinking a cup of chamomile tea. If you cannot sleep after lying in bed for more than half an hour, get up and do something monotonous like reading or ironing. Then, when you feel sleepy, go to bed.
- Not eating a heavy meal or drinking a lot before bedtime. Stay away from caffeine found in coffee, tea, chocolate and soda. Alcohol isn't a good idea either. Besides disrupting your sleep, alcohol can trigger PMS symptoms.
- Taking magnesium tablets. Some women find magnesium helps them to sleep better. It is often called nature's own tranquillizer and, as we saw earlier, it helps relieve PMS symptoms too.
- Using visualization techniques. This can help if you find it hard to switch off from the day's events. Focus your mind on something that is relaxing, your dream location or happy memories, and you may find it easier to let go of the day.

- Practising relaxation techniques. Try lying on your back in bed, tensing every part of your body in turn, and then relaxing each bit. This way, you can actually feel how good it is to relax. You might want to do this with relaxing music playing in the background.
- Adding aromatherapy oils, such as lavender or bergamot, to your bath. Or sprinkle a few drops of lavender essential oil on your pillow or have a gentle massage with the oils. As we have already seen, herbs can help with sleep problems. Valerian, hops, passionflower, chamomile and skullcap all work as gentle sedatives and can improve the quality and duration of sleep.
- Avoiding long daytime naps, which can cause fragmented sleep or insomnia. Making love can also help you to go to sleep by relaxing you and releasing tension.
- About an hour before you go to bed, writing a 'to do' list for tomorrow and putting out the clothes you want to wear. This stops you mulling over what you need to do, and wear, the next day.

And if none of the above work, try not to worry and to keep things in perspective. The more you get anxious about not getting a good night's sleep, the less likely you are to sleep at all. And the chances are that if you don't sleep well one night, you'll sleep like a log the next, especially if you are doing your daily exercise and practising the stress-busting tips in this chapter.

11
Five alternative therapies for PMS

Diet, exercise and stress reduction are the backbone of natural therapy for PMS, but there are a number of other alternatives[23] or natural therapies that may be able to help. Bear in mind, though, that alternative therapies are a complement to the natural healing of PMS, and they won't be able to help you much if you are not eating correctly, exercising properly and watching your stress levels.

Herbal supplements have already been discussed in this book. Yoga was mentioned in Chapter 5, and light therapy will be explored in the next chapter. Here are five other approaches recognized for their ability to ease PMS:

Massage

A good massage can be soothing, relaxing and stimulating – and extremely beneficial when your symptoms are getting the better of you. But stress relief is not the only benefit of massage. Other benefits include improved circulation and metabolism, lowered blood pressure, increased levels of endorphins, improved sleep and relief from pain.

For PMS, the most helpful kind of massage is probably Swedish massage. The skin and muscles are gently stroked with extra pressure being given on tight, knotted areas. To work on specific areas that are causing tension, you may want to try shiatsu, which involves pressure placed on various points of your body to break up and release energy blockages. Make sure the massage is comfortable; if it feels too rough or doesn't make you feel good, tell the masseur or masseuse – he or she will welcome the feedback.

Or try some DIY massage techniques:
* *Every morning and evening, hammer out the kinks.* Using your fists, gently thump the outside of your body, starting with your legs and arms, working from top to bottom. Then move inwards to your torso and thump from bottom to top. When done before bed, this calms the mind and beats out the stress and tension of the day.

One warning: If you are taking any kind of blood thinner, such as Coumadin (warfarin), avoid this one; you could end up with bruising.

- *Rub your abdomen after every meal.* Most of us do this instinctively, especially after overeating. Place one or both palms on your abdomen and rub it in clockwise circles. This is the same direction that food naturally moves through your intestine, so your circular massage will help to stimulate digestion.

- *Give your hands a massage every day.* You can do this whenever you put on hand cream. Start with the bottoms of your palms by clasping your fingers and rubbing the heels of your palms together in a circular motion. Then, with your hands still clasped, take one thumb and massage the area just below your other thumb in a circular motion, moving outwards to the centre of the palm. Repeat with the other hand. Then release your fingers and use your thumbs and index fingers to knead your palms, wrists and the webbing between your fingers. With one hand, gently pull each finger of the other hand. Finish by using your thumb and index finger to pinch the webbing between your other thumb and index finger.

- *Hold the side of your head to help relieve tension.* Use the full hand and press gently with your palms, just above your ears and with your fingers meeting in the middle of your forehead; then let go. It is actually the sensation of pressure and then letting go that is relaxing. Pressure should be light since the aim is to hold, not press.

- *Roll on a tennis ball whenever you feel tense/tight muscles.* If your foot feels tense, stand with one hand against a wall for support and place the arch of one foot on top of the ball. Gradually add more body weight over the foot, allowing the ball to press into your arch. Begin to slowly move your foot, allowing the ball to massage your heel, forefoot and toes. You can also lie on the ball to get at that hard-to-reach spot between the shoulder blades or to soothe tension in your lower back. For tight hips, sit on the ball, wiggling your bottom around and holding it in any spot that feels particularly beneficial.

Acupuncture and acupressure

Acupuncture is part of the Chinese practice of medicine that involves using fine needles to regulate the flow of energy (called chi) in the body, stimulate the body's own healing responses, and remove blockages of energy flow that may be triggering symptoms. The application of heat and massage may also be part of the process. Many women with PMS find acupuncture is helpful for relieving symptoms and boosting energy. In acupressure, instead of using needles to change the energy flow, the practitioner applies pressure to various body parts. Shiatsu is another practice that involves the application of pressure to energy pathways.

Aromatherapy

Aromatherapy oils are essential oils extracted from aromatic plants. Each essential oil works through your sense of smell and by being absorbed by the skin and lungs into your bloodstream, where it has a healing and relaxing effect on organs, glands and tissues. With the exception of lavender and tea tree, essential oils should be blended with carrier oil, such as almond oil, or diluted in water before coming into contact with your skin. Drops of essential oil can also be used directly in your bath or used as massage oil. Some oils are not appropriate during pregnancy: check with a qualified practitioner before using any oil if you think you may be pregnant.

The aromatherapy oils typically prescribed by aromatherapists for general PMS symptoms include: chamomile, clary sage, geranium, lavender, melissa, rose, rosemary and sandalwood. For bloating or breast tenderness, try: juniper, grapefruit, lemon, geranium and lavender. For general irritability, use: bergamot, geranium, clary sage. For sadness and depression, try: basil, bergamot, clary sage, geranium, jasmine, lavender, neroli, rose. For cramps: lavender, clary sage, chamomile. For fatigue: rosemary and basil to stimulate and energize; lavender and marjoram to encourage rest at the end of the day. For headaches: basil, chamomile, lavender, melissa, rose, rosemary, peppermint. For insomnia: basil, chamomile, juniper, lavender, sandalwood, ylang ylang. For anxiety or nervous tension: bergamot, camphor, chamomile, lavender, melissa.

Pheromones

It has been suggested that regular sex can help reduce PMS symptoms. American reproductive biologist Winifred Cutler believes that for heterosexual women this is due to the effect of smelling a man's pheromones. Women in her trials reported that after three months of smelling their partner's armpits, periods were more regular and PMS reduced. Do bear in mind, though, that it has to be the same armpits that you are sniffing nightly – apparently different pheromones don't have the same normalizing effect on your hormones! Orgasms are well known for helping to relieve period pain and cramps, and for relieving stress, anxiety and low moods.

Homeopathy

Homeopathy is based on the concept of like cures like in the same way that vaccinations work. The homeopath believes that physical symptoms such as PMS are the result of certain emotional or physical disturbances and he or she will decide on a remedy that will suit you best. Research[24] suggests that homeopathic treatments can be of benefit to women with PMS, but if you are interested in homeopathy don't try to treat yourself. Instead, visit a qualified practitioner. Homeopathic remedies often prescribed for PMS include nux vomica for irritability and food cravings, natrum mur for fluid retention, pulsatilla for feeling tearful, and sepia for irritability and depression.

Reflexology

Reflexologists believe that points on your hands and feet correspond to various organs and systems in your body, and that pressing on them can correct imbalances. Reflexology has been shown to help women with PMS. In one study, pressure in the correct places was applied to women in one group and in the incorrect places for women in another. The women who had the real reflexology showed a significant improvement in symptoms. When a reflexologist treats you for PMS using special thumb and finger techniques, he or she will pay particular attention to areas in your feet that correspond to the pelvis and female organs. Many women say that at the end of a session they feel as relaxed as if they have had a full body massage.

Note: If you do want to experiment with complementary therapies, check with your doctor first if you are pregnant or hoping to be; or are on medication or have a pre-existing medical condition. Complementary therapies are those not typically prescribed by medical doctors, but any treatment you try has the potential to be dangerous if used improperly. So make sure that the therapist you visit is qualified, beware of any treatment with an outrageous price tag, and avoid any quick-fix treatments that offer to cure PMS.

12

Light up your life

When you are trying to beat PMS, it is worth thinking about something as simple and natural as light. Have you ever noticed how much happier you feel when it is a bright, sunny day? You feel energized and eager to live it up. In contrast, think about how you feel when the clocks go back and the days get gloomier and shorter and night-time falls depressingly early.

Light, or the lack of daylight, may affect your emotional and physical health far more than you realize. The condition called SAD (seasonal affective disorder) is a well-known seasonal depression that hits during the winter months and lifts during the spring and summer. Symptoms of SAD are often similar to PMS; people feel depressed and tired and crave sweet foods. And you may find that in the winter the lack of light makes your symptoms worse.

But why should PMS be connected to light? The answer is to do with your metabolic cycles, which are light dependent. Your sleep cycle is very much governed by the light or lack of it. When the sun goes down and darkness falls, your brain begins to produce a neurotransmitter called melatonin which makes you feel drowsy and prepares your body for sleep. When you are exposed to bright light, however, your brain starts to convert melatonin to serotonin which energizes you and makes you feel alert and confident. Melatonin and serotonin are two substances that can be easily converted from one to the other.

You want to have a plentiful supply of serotonin, not just because it makes you feel good, but also because it provides the raw material for melatonin so that you can fall asleep at night. Without enough serotonin you can end up feeling depressed and irritable, with food cravings, and you can also have problems sleeping. Sounds a bit like PMS, doesn't it?

If you think that low levels of serotonin and melatonin sound similar to signs of PMS, then you are right because research[25] has shown that serotonin/melatonin levels actually drop a little in order for ovulation to occur. This means you are susceptible to mood swings and food cravings in the run-up to your period. Clearly, too little serotonin and melatonin can play a big part in triggering PMS symptoms or making them worse, and there is something that can significantly decrease your levels of these neurotransmitters – lack of light.

The PMS–light connection

It is clear that too little serotonin and melatonin, as well as too little light, are related. Here is a checklist of the symptoms caused by both:

- a change of appetite
- irritability
- tendency to oversleep
- low self-esteem
- weight gain
- difficulty in concentrating
- fatigue or low energy levels
- reluctance to socialize

All these symptoms are also found in PMS; the lack of light triggers a lack of serotonin, which makes PMS worse. So if you have got PMS, one of the simplest and most effective natural therapies is to get some light into your life. By getting plenty of light you will increase your serotonin and melatonin levels, your mood will be lighter, and you will have more energy. This is especially important if your PMS tends to get worse in the winter or if you suffer from depression.

Light therapy

To boost your serotonin production you need to expose yourself either to full-spectrum light that you get from the sun or a bright white light. Incandescent lights that you may have in your lamps just aren't the same. If it is summer time or you live in a sunny climate, light therapy is simple. You just need to walk outdoors for about 30 minutes each day – preferably in the morning. Don't wear sunglasses or tinted contact lenses, or your eyes will not be exposed to the light rays. Raise your face to the sky, but don't look directly at the sun though. Even on a cloudy day, the sun provides the full spectrum of light that the body needs.

To help regulate the production of serotonin and melatonin it has been suggested that women with PMS and irregular periods should also try to eliminate all outside sources of light at night to get their body back to a proper dark and light cycle. This helps to orchestrate the correct timing of the secretion of melatonin and serotonin. It might be worth putting black-out curtains up to shut out street lights or perhaps to wear an eye mask to bed.

If you think you need something more to boost the production of serotonin/melatonin, you might want to think about a special light box that can provide fluorescent full-spectrum light, or a bright white light that contains no UV wavelengths because they can cause skin cancer. There are also new systems that use cool-white and bi-axial lamps. The light is measured in units called lux and a typical light box provides 10,000 lux. Daylight is approximately 5,000 lux and it takes about 2,500 lux to have a therapeutic effect on your internal clock.

Scientists believe that bright-light therapy works by suppressing daytime elevation of the hormone melatonin (a substance that promotes sleep), and increasing the amount of mood-elevating brain chemical serotonin. Interestingly, these changes in neurotransmitters can reduce carbohydrate cravings and the need for an inordinate amount of sleep – which are both hallmarks of PMS and depression. Studies also show that bright-light therapy can also be effective for insomnia, helping to restore normal sleep patterns in people who cannot fall asleep at night or who wake up too early in the morning (there are dawn/dusk simulators sold by light-box companies for this purpose).

Light therapy has also been used to successfully treat the depression associated with PMS, chronic anxiety and panic attacks, severe jet lag, and eating disorders such as anorexia nervosa and bulimia. You can do light therapy yourself as long as you follow to the letter the instructions with your box and don't overdo it – but it is always best to check with your doctor first for advice. The downside of light therapy is that sometimes it can take a long time; those with SAD may need to sit in front of a lamp both for a few hours in the morning and the evening in the winter months. That is not easy to do, and some experts have suggested that those with

SAD should replace their ordinary light bulbs with full-spectrum versions so they can get a good blast during the day.

What you can expect

Before you use light therapy for PMS, depression or for any other ailment, you should talk to your doctor. (Indeed, if you suffer from any type of depression, you should be under a doctor's care.) When being outdoors is not an available option, the most common way to receive light therapy is to use a light box fitted with a white or full-spectrum light. Many users report that full-spectrum light, which simulates daylight, is more pleasant for the eye than white light, although there is no difference in the benefits received. Many full-spectrum lights now eliminate the skin-damaging ultraviolet (UV) rays.

For a treatment, the light box (which is small enough to be set on a table) should be placed where it is level with the eyes. Follow the manufacturer's instructions regarding where you should sit for optimum results. You may read, eat, or do other activities during the session. Depending on the brightness of the light source, treatment can take anywhere from 15 minutes to three hours. If you would rather move around during your treatment, you may prefer to use a light visor, which is worn on the head (like a tennis visor) and powered with rechargeable batteries. Because light visors are worn so close to the eyes, although they typically have a maximum of just 3,000 lux, treatment sessions do not necessarily take longer.

Cautions: Check with a health-care professional before starting any form of light therapy. If you have glaucoma, cataracts or retinal detachment, check with your doctor before starting light therapy. Never look directly into the light source during your therapy. If you have a rash accompanied by a fever, talk to your doctor before starting light therapy (you may have an infection such as measles or chicken pox). If your skin or eyes are highly sensitive to light, avoid light therapy. Avoid light therapy if you have any type of bipolar disorder (e.g. manic depression).

Supplementing with melatonin?

Supplementing with melatonin may help in some cases, but for most of us it is not necessary. Adding melatonin as a drug is not the answer as it is a short cut that does not address the root cause of the problem. As always, the best way to encourage your body to regulate the melatonin/serotonin cycle is to avoid quick fixes and to eat healthily, take care of your body through exercise and relaxation, and get plenty of quality sleep, fresh air and natural light.

13

You are what you think

Negative thinking, anger, irritation, frustration and anxiety can all encourage your body to produce stress hormones, in particular cortisol and, as we have seen earlier, cortisol can use up your progesterone supply and make your symptoms worse. By contrast, positive thinking, laughter, happiness and joy can all reduce stress – and anything that helps to reduce stress is good news if you have got PMS.

The power of positive thinking

Research[26] shows that people who are more optimistic about life feel healthier and happier, and women who think positively about themselves and their lives are more likely to do well in combating PMS than those who feel that their lives are out of control.[27]

In study after study, placebos have 'cured' a large number and variety of diseases, from headaches to cancer. No one is really sure how or why this can happen, but some experts believe it is because they tap into the patient's expectations of getting better. If patients believe a medicine really will help, they tend to get better. That is because positive thoughts can literally rearrange body chemistry, lower the production of stress hormones, and increase the production of endorphins and other feel-good chemicals. In short, placebos prove that good thoughts really can boost health and well-being.

You do not need to be prescribed a placebo to feel the benefits of positive thinking. You can start right now by thinking uplifting thoughts. Try to focus on what you have to be grateful for in your life. Think about things that make you smile and remember the successes you have had in your life. Appreciate the joy in ordinary things, the beauty of nature and the goodness of the people around you. Spend time with people that you love, and as much as possible do the things you love. Look for things to be happy about. A complement to positive thinking is to let go of negative thoughts when they strike. Cancel them out with positive ones or simply let them go.

Laughter really is the best medicine. Try not to forget that positive thinking is a natural therapy you can use at any time, anywhere, for whatever it is that is troubling you. There is no correct way to practise the natural therapy of positive thinking – you need to find out what works best for you – but hopefully the suggestions in this chapter will encourage you to think good thoughts whenever possible.

The best medicine

Positive self-talk

Studies show[28] that when women with PMS feel good about themselves, they feel happier – and when they feel happier, their symptoms ease. Positive thinking can have a therapeutic effect on your symptoms, but far too many of us talk negatively to ourselves. Do you say things like: 'I'm stupid'; 'I always mess things up'; 'It's bound to go wrong'; and 'I'm no good at that'?

If you talk negatively about yourself, it will not be long before you start agreeing with yourself. So, the next time you catch yourself thinking or talking negatively, try using something positive instead. Replace 'I can't' with 'I'll try' or 'I'll do my best'. Replace 'I'm no good' with 'I learn from mistakes'. Replace 'I'm useless' with 'I can learn'. Replace 'It's only me' with 'It's me and I'm a terrific person'. Even if you don't believe it, try this exercise.

When you say positive things to yourself, what you are doing is retraining your mind. It is almost like learning a new language. The words and phrases come before the understanding. It is a struggle at first, and it will take time and patience and constant repetition, but then you start to see the bigger picture. Believing the positive things you say about yourself will eventually come. For now, just keep telling yourself positive things over and over again. Start reprogramming your mind. It may help to create a list of positive affirmations such as 'I value myself' or 'I deserve to be happy' or 'I can handle this'. Keep these affirmations in the present tense, and keep them positive. Practise saying them all the time.

Be your own best friend

This technique is really great when negative thoughts start to overwhelm you. How do you talk to yourself? Are you kind and considerate, or are you harsh and judgemental? If your best friend called you and wanted reassuring, would you use negative words and tell her she was no good? No, you would offer comfort and support. Why not do the same for yourself? When things get tough, become your own best friend. Imagine that you have stepped outside of your body and that you are standing by yourself. Now hold your hand. What would you say that was reassuring and comforting? How would you help this person to feel better about herself? Would you tell her that she is doing well and that she has lots of good qualities and that good things lie ahead? Talk to yourself in the way you would to a best friend or loved one who was feeling down.

Create success for yourself

Find a comfortable place, close your eyes, and relax. Follow your breathing and then see your success in action. Picture the scene that you would like to create. See yourself being successful, happy and positive about life. You look confident and relaxed. Feel what it is like to be a success. See people treating you with the respect you deserve. Make this vision as real as you can. See and hear the whole thing in colour, create the sound effects, feel the reality of your success. When you are ready, let your thoughts return, open your eyes, and come back to the room. (If during this exercise negative thoughts are getting the better of you, imagine them floating away like a balloon. Let your balloon go and never think about it again.)

Stop comparing yourself

Do you ever feel that you are not as good, clever or attractive as someone else? Each time you compare yourself with other people, you are mistrusting yourself. The next time you find yourself comparing yourself with others, tell yourself that you are unique. Accept and make the most of your differences. They are what make you a unique and original person with your own special place in the world.

Don't believe everything you feel

Just because you feel something does not mean it is true. For example, PMS can make you feel terrible, but this does not mean you *are* terrible. You are the one in charge of your feelings, not the other way round.

Don't take it personally

When you have PMS, the world tends to shrink. Everything seems to revolve around you and the way you feel. Something goes wrong, and it is your fault. Your partner works late, and it is because he wants to get away from you. Stop thinking that everything revolves around you. Lots of things have nothing to do with you. People have other things going on in their lives apart from you.

Discover the positives

There is a positive side to almost everything, even PMS. One 1989 study at the Canadian Well Woman clinic revealed that seven out of ten women did have at least one positive symptom in their premenstrual phase. The study showed that women are very sensitive during this time to lights, sounds and smells, and that women who were creative – artists, actresses, musicians – reported that they felt more creative and inspired. Some 31 per cent of the women in the Canadian study even reported an increased enjoyment of sex.

Stop exaggerating

PMS is likely to make you take the negative in a situation and blow it up out of all proportion. Focusing on just the negative is unrealistic and unfair. Yes, you had an argument with your partner, but most of the time you get on really well. Yes, you had a problem at work, but this does not mean you cannot do your job. Yes, the kids can be a nightmare sometimes and you lose your temper, but most of the time you are a great mum. The next time you feel low, pay attention to your thinking patterns. You do not need to replace negative thoughts with positive ones all the time. You just need to replace them with more realistic, balanced ones. But fortunately a realistic outlook is often much more optimistic than a negative one because realistic thoughts take into account both the negative and the positive, whereas negative thoughts just focus on the negative.

Focus on your strengths

When you feel low, lift yourself up by focusing on your strengths. Write down as many as you can think of. Be proud of yourself. Self-respect opens the door to optimism. Appreciate the depth and variety of your personality. If you do feel low when PMS strikes, remind yourself that you also have a bright side to your personality. Those low moments are part of the interesting, complex woman that you are.

14

A to Z of common symptoms and natural ways to treat them

If you have been eating healthily, exercising regularly and taking care of yourself according to the advice given in the previous chapters, you may find that your body reaches a state of good health and your symptoms disappear after two or three months. If, however, you find that some symptoms still surface from time to time, the following A to Z of the most common symptoms experienced by women with PMS, and natural ways to treat them, should help.

Note: For herbal remedies for specific symptoms, you may also want to refer to the advice given in Chapter 7.

Aches and pains

You may find that you get stiffness, pain or tenderness in the back, neck or joints in the run-up to your period. This pain is not related to an underlying disorder, such as arthritis, and typically resolves when your period arrives. A major cause is hormonal fluctuations, and it may be exacerbated by poor diet and stress. The following recommendations should help:

- Try a heat pad or soak in a warm bath for 30 minutes to increase the blood flow to the muscles.
- Avoid physically demanding activities for a few days and substitute stretching or gentle yoga for high-impact exercise. Perform low-impact exercise as well as stretching to condition your back, joints and muscles, and over time this should decrease premenstrual discomfort.
- Try to avoid over-the-counter painkillers unless absolutely necessary. Capsaicin creams may prove useful if they are applied several times a day. Capsaicin, a component of chilli peppers, blocks the bio-chemicals that cause pain.
- Pay attention to your posture – including how you sit, stand or carry items – and try to reduce the strain on your back and neck.

When standing, keep your head held high, your pelvis forward, and your abdomen and buttocks tucked in. When sitting, keep your spine against the back of the chair and your knees a little higher than your hips. When carrying items, remember that heavy bags put pressure on your back, so try to alter the load.

- If you have regular severe back and neck pain that does not come and go with your menstrual cycle, consult your doctor for recommendations and back-strengthening exercises.

Acne, spots and problem skin

Blackheads, whiteheads, pustules and cysts often appear on the face in the premenstrual period, even in adult women. Spots and pimples can also occur on your back, neck and buttocks. According to Anthony Chu, senior dermatologist at the Imperial College of Science, Technology and Medicine, Hammersmith Hospital in London, the cause of spots is not chocolate, fatty food, cakes, sweets or poor hygiene, although these things won't help the condition. Instead, the cause is an increase in the skin's production of oil, called sebum. Oestrogen helps to regulate sebum, but in the run-up to your period oestrogen levels fall and more sebum is produced. Androgen hormones – of which testosterone is the most well known – increase the production of sebum. In women who get spots only in the run-up to a period, it is thought that for some reason the adrenal glands may be producing too much of the hormone called androgen.

The typical treatment offered for spots is antibiotics, but this is not a good idea if you have PMS as it will not help to address the real cause of the problem. If you do suffer from bouts of premenstrual spots, keep your blood sugar levels in balance and control stress levels so that your adrenal glands can function normally. Although there is no known cure for premenstrual acne, the following remedies may help to keep the blemishes under control:

- It is especially important that you include plenty of phytoestrogens in your diet (see p. 19). Phytoestrogens can help your body control the amount of testosterone circulating in your blood.
- Vitamin B6[29] has been shown to be beneficial for spots caused by PMS. Foods rich in B6 include bananas, fish, lean meat, nuts, seeds and wholegrains.

- Make sure you get your essential fatty acids. Flaxseed oil and primrose oil are good sources of the essential fatty acids needed to keep skin smooth and clear.
- While there is no known relationship between specific foods and acne flare-ups, if you notice any dietary triggers for acne, avoid these foods. You should also limit your intake of alcohol, sugar, processed food, salt, butter, caffeine, chocolate, eggs, fried foods, meat, margarine, wheat, soft drinks and food containing hydrogenated vegetable oils.
- To ease inflammation or prevent infection, eat lots of garlic. Garlic is a powerful antibiotic. Grate it on to your food or take it as a supplement every day.
- Women with PMS can be deficient in zinc, which is important for hormonal balance. It is also helpful for keeping testosterone and acne flare-ups in check. Make sure you are getting enough zinc in your diet, found in foods such as shellfish, soya beans and sunflower and pumpkin seeds. You may also want to take 30 mg a day of a zinc supplement for two to three months.
- Sulphur-rich foods such as eggs, onion and live yogurt with bifidus and acidophilus bacteria help to rebalance the bacteria in your gut and can protect against skin inflammation.
- Regular exercise is helpful because it encourages hormonal balance and healthy blood flow to your face to help flush out toxins.
- Keep make-up to a minimum and cleanse thoroughly with a mild but not astringent skincare product. Never leave make-up on at night and choose oil-free moisturizers and foundations. Opt for loose rather than pressed powders, and powder blushes instead of creams. Look for the word 'non-comedogenic' on labels. Always try to cleanse your skin twice a day, but don't use harsh cleansers or toners with alcohol as these strip the skin of natural oils, encouraging it to produce more in response, and increase the chance of spots.
- Avoid abrasive scrubs. They do not remove dead skin, but they can cause infection and make acne worse. Use one specifically recommended by a dermatologist if you use one at all.
- Never pick or squeeze spots – this can cause scarring.
- Tea tree oil has good antiseptic, anti-bacterial and anti-fungal properties. Use it to dab on to your spots. A study conducted by the Department of Dermatology of the Royal Prince Alfred

Hospital in New South Wales, Australia, found a 5 per cent solution of tea tree oil was as effective as a 5 per cent solution of benzoyl peroxide for most cases of acne, and had no side-effects. You may want to use a tea tree moisturizer.

- Ketsugo is made from isolutrol, a substance originally derived from shark's bile, but now synthesized. It is rich in antioxidants and, according to Dr David Fenton from St John's Department of Dermatology at St Thomas's Hospital in London, it appears to be able to regulate the production of sebum and soften the skin.
- Pure aloe vera gel is anti-bacterial and soothing. Some women find that dabbing it on their acne every day really helps.
- For angry inflamed spots or acne, witch hazel is cooling and soothing. Dab directly on the acne. Echinacea is one of nature's most powerful antibiotics. Dab a tincture or cream on the affected skin daily.
- If your doctor tells you that you have higher than normal androgen levels, the herb saw palmetto can work as an anti-androgen and this can be helpful for premenstrual acne. Perhaps the most helpful herb, though, is agnus castus (chasteberry; see p. 49) which has been found to be beneficial in the treatment of PMS acne. Other beneficial herbs include burdock root, red clover and milk thistle, which are powerful blood cleansers. All these should be prescribed by a medical herbalist.
- Light therapy, which involves shining different types of light on the acne, can help. Red lights have been shown to open capillaries and boost circulation while blue light closes them. Ask a dermatologist for advice.
- Dermatitis or eczema, both of which can cause itching, can also occur in the run-up to a period. Itching typically occurs on the hands, face, scalp and behind the knees, and it can increase with stress so watch your stress levels. First check that you don't have any allergic reaction to the food you are eating or the substances that come into contact with your skin, such as washing powder. Then consider these remedies to reduce your discomfort:
  – Try using a cortisone cream or lotion or a calamine-type lotion.
  – Cool compresses, or a washcloth soaked in milk and water, can help.
  – Itchy skin is known to get worse with stress, so why not try a relaxing massage.
  – Apply cooled chamomile tea to the skin with a soft cloth.

– Avoid scratching, and use breathing and relaxation strategies when the urge strikes.
– Keep your fingernails short, smooth and clean.
– Evening primrose oil may be able to relieve the itchiness associated with dry skin.
– Known mainly for its relaxing effects used for anxiety and insomnia, some herbal specialists prescribe oral lavender for dry skin conditions.

Bloating

The hormonal fluctuations that occur just before your period can cause your kidneys to retain water and salt, and this is what makes you feel bloated and heavy. The area under your eyes may also appear puffy, and again this is due to temporary water retention. Over-the-counter remedies are not advised as they can leach valuable nutrients from your body, but if you do get fluid retention, there are a number of things you can do to help yourself:

• Cut down on your salt intake. Use less salt in your cooking, watch out for hidden salts in your food, and look for other ways to enhance flavour – for example, using herbs and spices instead.
• Increase your fluid intake. You need to drink more, not less, to help your body dilute the salt in your tissues and allow you to excrete more salt and fluid. Aim to drink at least two to three litres of water a day.
• Reduce the amount of caffeine in your diet. Caffeine is a diuretic, but it won't ease bloating because it hinders the secretion of excess salt and toxins from your body.
• Make sure that your diet includes sufficient B vitamins, especially Vitamin B6, found in bananas, lean meat, fish, nuts, seeds and wholegrains, which is a tried and tested remedy for PMS water retention.
• Eat foods that naturally decrease fluid retention, like asparagus, cider vinegar, alfalfa sprouts and dandelion flowers. And eat more potassium-rich food to bring down your body's sodium level as the two minerals balance each other out. Reach for those bananas, apricots, black beans, lentils, tomatoes, green leafy vegetables and fresh fruits.

- Keep your blood sugar levels in balance. When blood sugar levels drop, adrenaline is released to move sugar quickly from your cells into your blood. When the sugar leaves the cells it is replaced by water, which contributes to that bloated feeling.
- Get moving. Moderate exercise will make you sweat and hasten the transport of water through your body.
- Studies at the University of Reading have shown the surprising effectiveness of colladeen, a mix of grapeseed extract, bilberry and cranberry extract, for the relief of PMS bloating.
- Aromatherapy oils can be helpful in easing bloating. Add fennel or chamomile to a warm bath and soak for 20 minutes for the best effect. You may also want to use juniper as a massage oil.
- Dandelion and parsley are natural herbal diuretics packed with PMS-beating nutrients that allow fluid to be released without losing nutrients.
- Elevate your feet if you are prone to swelling in the ankles. And wear support stockings/tights to ease discomfort.
- Bloating may be the result of constipation, so refer to the section on digestive problems below.

Breast tenderness

Breast swelling and pain in the week or so before your period are normal reactions to fluctuating hormone levels. You may find it hard to hug or sleep because you cannot find a comfortable position. If you suffer from breast tenderness, make sure you wear a comfortable supportive bra – one that does not irritate the nipple area as you move. Then try the recommendations below:

- Studies[30] have shown that women who live in Asian countries do not have the same degree of breast discomfort, and diet is the crucial factor here. The diet of most Asian women tends to be based less on processed and fatty food. So the first step is to eat healthily according to the 12-week plan.
- Make sure you get your phytoestrogens, found in foods such as soya products, chickpeas and lentils. The diet of Asian women is high in phytoestrogens, which help keep their hormones in balance.
- Cut down on foods and drinks containing caffeine. They have been shown to increase problems related to tender breasts.

- Increase your fibre intake. Research[31] has shown that there may be a link between constipation and a painful breast condition called fibrocystic breast disease. So make sure you drink enough water and have a good intake of fibre to ensure bowel regularity. You may also like to sprinkle some linseeds on your cereal in the morning. Don't, however, include bran in your diet. Bran can make things worse because it contains substances called phylates which can interfere with the absorption of important PMS-beating nutrients, like magnesium and calcium.
- Vitamin E has been shown[32] to reduce breast pain and tenderness in many studies. Eat foods rich in Vitamin E, such as oats, sunflower oil, wholegrains, soya oil and dark-green leafy vegetables. You may also want to take a supplement for a couple of months to give you a kick start.
- Eat some live yogurt every day. Breast tenderness may be related to an excess of oestrogen, and the beneficial bacteria in live yogurt can help to reabsorb old hormones and also to increase the efficiency of your bowel movements.
- Increase your intake of omega 3 fatty acids. Omega 3 fatty acids, found in fish oil, have been found to relieve breast tenderness and fluid retention. Take fish oil capsules or eat more fish, or sprinkle linseeds and hemp seeds on to your salads and soups.
- The B vitamins are of particular value if you suffer from breast tenderness because they help your liver break down excess oestrogen. Improve your intake of B vitamin foods, and think about taking a B complex supplement for a couple of months.
- Older studies[33] showed that supplementing your diet with evening primrose oil that contains GLA (gamma linolenic acid) could reduce breast discomfort, although more recent studies have not backed this up. The suggested dosage is between 240 mg and 320 mg a day. Do bear in mind, though, that evening primrose oil needs to be taken for about three months to be effective, so you need to be patient.
- A number of essential aromatherapy oils, such as lavender, fennel and juniper, can encourage lymphatic drainage and relieve breast pain by helping to regulate hormones. Massage them on to your breasts, putting one drop of your chosen oil in a teaspoonful of carrier oil such as sweet almond or sunflower, or use a few drops in your bath.
- The herb ginkgo biloba has proved to be effective according to

one French study[34] where women with PMS breast tenderness taking ginkgo biloba reported less pain than those taking a placebo. Other helpful herbs include agnus castus (chasteberry) to balance hormones and milk thistle to help your liver to process oestrogen efficiently, allowing any excess to be excreted. Ask a medical herbalist for advice.

Note: You might also consider taking a non-prescription pain reliever such as aspirin and ibuprofen. Most breast pain is not linked to severe health conditions, like cancer, but never ignore the pain. Any unusual changes should be reported to your doctor.

Cramps

Premenstrual cramps or pain in the pelvic region, abdomen, back or thighs are thought to be due to an excess of prostaglandins, the hormones that stimulate the uterus. If you are prone to severe cramps you might initially consider a non-prescription pain reliever such as aspirin and ibuprofen. You should also try the following recommendations:

- Apply heat with a hot water bottle or a heat pad or immerse yourself in a hot bath.
- Increase your intake of essential oils. Omega 3 fatty acids found in fish oil have been found to relieve painful periods, and gamma linolenic acid found in evening primrose oil can ease premenstrual breast tenderness and pelvic cramps. Take a fish oil supplement or increase your intake of fish. For optimal absorption, these essential fatty acids require that Vitamin E be taken with them, so check that your multivitamin and mineral supplement contains enough Vitamin E. If you are vegetarian, take some hemp or flaxseed oil.
- Massage can relieve pain and muscle tension, including the discomfort of premenstrual cramps.
- If your pain is debilitating, consult your doctor to make sure you have not got an underlying pelvic or uterine problem.

Digestive problems

Digestive problems, such as diarrhoea, constipation and nausea, may occur in the run-up to a period. The most effective natural remedy is a healthy, fibre-rich diet, but the following may also help:

- Make sure you drink plenty of water. Drinking hot water with lemon juice in the morning will encourage regular bowel movements and ease constipation.
- Peppermint and fennel teas after a meal can ease digestion and reduce trapped wind.
- If you have diarrhoea, avoid alcohol, caffeine, milk and dairy products until the diarrhoea has subsided. Try some potassium-rich banana, apple sauce, rice and dry toast until you feel better to help restore balance to your body. You can also use live yogurt to replace beneficial bacteria in your intestines. Do not take any anti-diarrhoea medications until you have given these other recommendations a chance to work.
- Chew your food slowly and thoroughly to encourage proper digestion. Before you begin a meal, start with a few deep breaths and breathe fully as you eat. Try to avoid distractions when you eat, like the television.
- If you have intestinal cramping and wind all month long in spite of these remedies, you may have irritable bowel syndrome. This is a disorder that needs medical attention.
- If you get nausea along with digestive distress, try drinking chamomile tea three times a day. Vitamin B6 can help quell nausea. Increase the amount in your diet or take a supplement.
- Ginger is also great for easing nausea. Brew a cup of ginger tea and drink daily. If stomach acid is a problem, a cup of liquorice root tea has been shown to be effective.
- Acupressure has been found to be effective for reducing nausea. You can purchase acupressure bands to be worn around your wrists in many chemists.

Check out persistent symptoms with your doctor.

Disorientation and clumsiness

You may feel more accident-prone in the run-up to your period and there is a reason for this. Studies[35] show that in the premenstrual period, the nervous system is affected and this can cause lack of co-ordination, poor concentration and clumsiness. Difficulty in concentrating and becoming absent-minded may be related to fluid retention, lack of sleep and stress. The following natural therapies should help:

- Pay particular attention to eating little and often and cut down on caffeine to ensure that your nervous system isn't being over-worked by too much adrenaline.
- Make sure that your diet is sufficient in B vitamins – especially Vitamin B5 found in food such as wholegrains, whole brown rice, wholemeal bread, legumes, broccoli and tomatoes. Vitamin B5 is essential for optimum functioning of your nervous system. If lack of co-ordination is a real problem, you may want to take a supplement of 50 mg of Vitamin B5 a day, in addition to your usual multivitamin and mineral supplement.
- Ensure that your diet is sufficient in magnesium, which can help to control the stress response. Food sources include wheatbran, wheatgerm, nuts, flour, dark-green leafy vegetables, dried apricots, fish and tofu. The recommended dosage for the relief of PMS is 200–600 mg.
- Decrease your intake of stimulants such as caffeine, nicotine and sugar.
- Learn a relaxation technique to give your nervous system a chance to repair and relax. Just a few minutes a day of relaxation is enough.
- Try some essential oils to soothe your mind and body and reduce unhelpful stress. Melissa, lavender and chamomile all have a calming effect, which can help with problems that contribute to clumsiness.
- Your clumsiness and disorientation may simply be the result of fatigue or stress, and if this is the case, refer to the relevant sections in this book.

Concentration problems/poor memory

Some women find it hard to remember things or concentrate in the premenstrual phase. For example, you may need to read a page over and over again to get the sense of it or you may find yourself daydreaming when you need to be concentrating. If you start eating healthily, exercising regularly and finding ways to ease stress, you may find that this symptom disappears. You may also want to try one of the following:

- Research[36] has shown that ginkgo biloba can ease symptoms of PMS and also improve concentration, memory and reaction time. Ginkgo helps to deliver oxygen to your nerve cells and your brain.

If mental and/or physical disorientation is a problem, you may want to take a tincture of ginkgo for a period of three to four months. Remember, herbs take a few weeks of daily use to produce an improvement.

- Make sure your diet is sufficient in iron as low iron levels can be associated with memory problems and poor co-ordination.
- Practise yoga and meditation to help improve concentration and alertness. While you are doing your yoga you may want to silently and slowly count backwards from 100 once you are in a relaxed state as this will help stimulate circuitry in the brain. As your concentration improves, count back down from 200 or even 500.
- Inability to focus may be due to fluid retention, stress and lack of sleep, or even too much sleep, so you may want to refer to the relevant sections on sleep in this book.

Fatigue

Tiredness or fatigue is one of the most common symptoms reported by women with PMS; you may feel exhausted a few days before your period or experience mild fatigue throughout the entire premenstrual period. Insufficient amounts of serotonin may contribute to fatigue (and to sleep problems, which can exacerbate fatigue). Fatigue may also be caused by low blood sugar levels and water retention.

All the natural therapies given in this book should help boost your energy levels, but the following may be particularly helpful:

- Make sure you balance out your carbohydrate load with some low-fat protein to avoid the sugar highs and lows that cause fatigue. In fact, balancing your blood sugar levels is the best way to fight fatigue and boost your energy levels, so refer to the diet tips on balancing your blood sugar levels on p. 16.
- Step up your exercise routine, as women who exercise regularly tend to feel more energized than those who do not.
- Eat foods that are high in fatigue-fighting potassium and magnesium. Prime sources include fruit and dark-green leafy vegetables, nuts, seeds and beans. You also need to make sure you are getting enough iron-rich foods. Foods rich in iron include wheatgerm, dried fruit, shellfish, sardines, and red and dark-green fruits and vegetables. If you are a vegetarian, you may want to take kelp supplements.

- Refer to the recommendations for stress-busting and getting a good night's sleep given in Chapter 10 as stress and lack of sleep can all cause fatigue.
- If your fatigue persists, you may want to rule out candida (fungal overgrowth), anaemia and/or a food allergy, which can all get worse before a period.
- The B vitamins are crucial if you feel tired as one of the symptoms of a deficiency of the major B vitamins is lack of energy.
- Co-enzyme Q10, a substance present in all human tissue, is a vital catalyst for energy production, and if you are deficient in this you may feel tired. Food sources of co-enzyme Q10 include fish, organ meats (like liver, heart or kidney), and the germ portion of wholegrains. You may also want to take 30 mg a day of co-enzyme Q10 over a period of three months.
- Ginger can boost energy levels. Use it fresh in your food as a quick pick-me-up. Cinnamon is another energy-boosting spice.
- Aromatherapy oils such as basil and rosemary can be helpful in relieving mental and physical fatigue. Both are stimulating and renewing, and you may want to add a few drops to your bath or use in a vaporizer in your room.

Food cravings

Many women experience sugar and/or food cravings in the week leading up to their period. Under normal circumstances the advice would be self-restraint, but during the premenstrual period the cravings are biochemical urges triggered by your body to prevent drops in blood sugar. It also seems that during the premenstrual period, fluctuating blood sugar levels and fluctuating female hormones make the cravings even more intense.

The best and most effective way to control sugar and food cravings is to make sure you are eating little and often as this will keep your blood sugar levels in balance. It is also a good idea to avoid foods containing sugar and caffeine. Eating good-quality carbohydrates with a good-quality protein, on a little-and-often basis, is the best way to stop your blood sugar from surging and dropping, and without those drops you will soon find that your cravings are under control.

As well as eating little and often and following the PMS diet guidelines to eliminate food cravings, the following natural remedies and therapies may be helpful:

Chromium

Chromium is especially helpful for controlling food cravings because it is an essential mineral for the metabolism of sugar. Chromium also helps to regulate appetite. Foods rich in chromium include liver, mushrooms, wholegrains and yeast; and if you are not diabetic, you may want to think about taking a supplement for a few months until the cravings disappear. If your multivitamin and mineral supplement does not contain enough chromium, make sure you are getting around 200 mcg of chromium a day.

Garcinia cambognia

You may also want to take garcinia cambognia (see p. 50).

If the DIY techniques listed above don't help, you may want to consider asking your doctor or a nutritionist for advice, or join a supervised dietary programme.

Headaches

Headaches are common in premenstrual women and the most usual sort are the tension-type headaches, characterized by a dull, steady pain across the head and neck. Another headache associated with PMS is the sinus headache, which may actually be a sign of water retention, another common feature of PMS. The migraine type may also occur, and this is characterized by throbbing pain, in addition to visual disturbances, nausea and vomiting that can last from a few hours to a few days. Nobody knows the cause of premenstrual headaches and migraines, but it is suggested that they are triggered by the low levels of oestrogen before menstruation. It is interesting to note that many women who get migraines stop having headaches when they become pregnant, so the link between headaches and hormonal change is clear.

The best solution in the long term is to eat the hormone- and blood-sugar-regulating diet recommended in Chapter 3. Missing meals or nutrients can trigger a headache whether you are premenstrual or not. The following recommendations may help:

- See if you can find a pattern or a trigger to your headaches. When you get a headache, note what you ate, when you ate, and how you felt when you ate. Perhaps you are sensitive to certain foods when you are premenstrual. Watch out especially for foods such as cheese, red wine, chocolate, citrus juice or fruit that contains tyramine, phenylethylamine and histamine, which can all trigger headaches. Unfortunately, symptoms often don't hit you immediately after eating these foods, so you need to keep a diary for several weeks to notice a pattern. Typical tension headache triggers include stress, fatigue, too much sleep, lack of exercise, and activities that require repetitive motion such as chewing gum or grinding teeth. Migraines can be triggered by certain foods and drinks, or they can be hormonally triggered by perimenopause or the use of oral contraceptives, lack of sleep, bright lights, weather changes, stress and strong smells.
- Magnesium helps your muscles to relax and a deficiency can trigger headaches. So make sure your diet includes foods such as dark-green leafy vegetables, nuts and seeds, dark (non-milk) chocolate, soya beans and wholegrains. One study[37] showed that women who took 300 mg of magnesium twice a day reported fewer headaches than those who did not.
- Make sure your diet is rich in essential fatty acids – especially omega 3. Another study[38] showed that those prone to migraine had a significant reduction in symptoms when they took omega 3 fish oils every day.
- It is best to avoid over-the-counter painkillers as many painkillers contain caffeine and you can also develop an intolerance to them.
- Learn to relax. By reducing muscle tension, you may be able to ward off a considerable number of headaches. Sit or lie down in a dark, quiet room for 20 minutes. Place an ice pack on your forehead. Tension headaches sometimes respond better to the application of heat.
- Regular exercise and stretching can prevent many tension headaches.
- Do your yoga breathing exercises to increase the flow of blood and oxygen and glucose to your brain and improve your circulation. See Chapter 5.
- Treat yourself to a neck, shoulder and head massage. Whether it is a traditional massage or acupressure, releasing physical tension and improving circulation can promote feelings of well-being and

even prevent headaches. Simply rubbing your temples can relieve pain.

• Putting an ice pack on the area where the pain is focused can reduce the blood flow, which in turn eases the pain. In some cases a warm bath can alleviate headaches, especially if an essential herb such as lavender is added. Other helpful oils include rosemary, which can stimulate blood supply to the head, and eucalyptus, which eases pain. Add a few drops to your bath or make up a massage oil to use in a neck and shoulder massage.

• Some women find that orgasm can help get rid of headaches as it opens up the blood vessels, whereas others find that it can bring on a headache. If you do get a post-coital headache, most will go away by themselves in a few minutes or hours.

• Use a blend of relaxing aromatherapy oils as a massage oil or add a few drops in your bath. Lavender, chamomile and rosemary can all ease pain.

• Many women find that acupuncture or homeopathy are useful treatments for headaches and migraines.

• If you have a tension headache and cannot go into a dark room to relax, put your hands around the back of your head and drop your chin on your chest. Press your chin down and hold for a minute. Then use your hands to turn your head to the right and hold for a minute. Then back to centre and hold for a minute, then to the left and then back to centre, again for a minute.

• One study[39] showed that 70 per cent of those who get migraine had less frequent attacks when taking the herb feverfew. The herb milk thistle may also be beneficial as milk thistle helps to improve liver function.

• Don't ignore headaches that occur over and over again. They could be a sign of an underlying health problem. If you have tried various DIY measures or your headaches become more intense or persistent, ask your doctor for advice.

Mood swings

One of the classic signs of low blood sugar is mood swings, so the best advice if you are prone to this symptom is to eat healthy and nutritious meals and snacks throughout the day. Don't go for long periods without food. And avoid caffeine and foods packed with sugar. Other helpful recommendations include:

- Consider taking a B vitamin supplement, magnesium supplement and omega 3 fish oil supplement in addition to your multivitamin and mineral supplement. The B vitamins can help your body to produce serotonin which is the 'feel-good' hormone. Magnesium is well known as 'nature's tranquillizer', and essential fatty acids are important for hormonal balance.
- Try some Siberian ginseng to help boost your adrenal glands and help you deal with stress.
- Try aromatherapy oils in a massage or a bath, such as relaxing lavender, mood-enhancing chamomile and rose oil, or calming sandalwood and clary sage.
- If you are prone to angry outbursts, remind yourself that you *do* have some control over yourself despite the way you are feeling. Question your motives. When you feel angry, stop and ask yourself why you feel this way and if your anger is appropriate to the situation. If you can do something positive, do it – but if you can't do anything, release your stress by using the stress-busting techniques in Chapter 10.

Mouth ulcers or cold sores

You may find that you are prone to mouth ulcers or cold sores in the run-up to your period. Although they may seem small, mouth ulcers and cold sores can be extremely painful and make it hard for you to eat, smile and laugh. They can also make you feel run down and tired. Nutritional deficiencies in iron, Vitamin B12 and folic acid have been linked to painful mouth ulcers. Vitamin C and zinc are also important because they can enhance immune function and aid wound healing. Other helpful strategies include:

- Good dental hygiene; it really is essential to floss every day.
- Eating plenty of salad with raw onions. Onions contain sulphur, which has healing properties.
- Avoiding sugar, citrus fruits and refined, processed foods. Also avoid chewing gum, lozenges, sharp sweets, mouthwashes, tobacco, coffee, citrus fruits and any other food that may trigger these sores.
- Paying attention to your stress levels – stress and allergies are perhaps the most common triggers for mouth ulcers and cold sores.

- You can buy gel-like ointment from your chemist – like Bonjela – that is applied directly to the mouth ulcer. It sticks to the sore and provides relief. If your ulcer or cold sore does not heal, consult your doctor.

Night sweats

Hot flushes or night sweats in the run-up to your period may not be linked to the approach of menopause but to PMS, because body temperature changes can sometimes be stimulated by the drop in ovarian hormones just before a period. Avoid alcohol, spicy foods and hot baths to minimize potential triggers and make sure you are eating healthily and exercising regularly. Make sure there is plenty of fresh air in your bedroom, that the temperature is set at around 65–78°F and bed linen is light, loose and cool. If the problem happens all month long and is accompanied by irregular periods, consult your doctor to see if they are related to the menopause.

15

Staying happy and healthy all month long

There is no instant cure for PMS and you need to commit yourself to at least two or three months of taking care of yourself according to the guidelines given in this book and finding what works best for you before you can really see the benefits.

If you find it hard to keep going or to stay motivated when things get tough, just imagine yourself a month or two from now having energy and no longer being at the mercy of your symptoms. Remind yourself that positive diet and lifestyle changes can not only ease your symptoms and make you look and feel better, they can also reduce your risk of premature ageing, obesity, heart disease, diabetes, osteoporosis and depression.

What greater motivation could there be than to feel happy and healthy not just all month long, but for the rest of your life!

Twelve golden rules

The 12 golden rules below will help keep you feeling great all month long, every month.

1 Keep track

Writing a symptom diary can help. Recognizing what is going on throughout the month by noting how you feel from day to day can help you schedule things to coincide with specific times. For example, if you tend to feel great for a few days during your cycle, that is the time to take your driving test, or go for a job interview, etc. If you know you may be feeling vulnerable on another day of your cycle, this is when you need to take it easy or tackle gentler tasks.

2 Keep your blood sugar levels balanced

The sweet cravings and mood swings that are often part of the PMS picture may be related to episodes of low blood sugar in the bloodstream. Three meals a day based on whole, unrefined foods, with healthy snacks such as fresh fruit and nuts in between, may prevent sugar lows, sweet cravings and help to regulate moods.

106

3 Eat plenty of fruit and vegetables

Fruit and vegetables are rich in PMS-beating hormone-balancing vitamins, minerals, antioxidants, fibre and phytoestrogens. Make sure you get at least five servings a day of vegetables and three of fruit.

4 Get your essential fats

Omega 6 oils found in nuts and seeds, evening primrose, sunflower oil and borage oil and omega 3 found in oily fish and flaxseed oil have a beneficial effect on your hormones, so make sure you include enough in your diet.

5 Drink plenty of water

Your body is around 70 per cent water so drink plenty (around six to eight glasses a day) to stay hydrated.

6 Take vitamins and minerals

Studies show that a lack of various nutrients can increase PMS symptoms. These nutrients include magnesium, calcium, Vitamin B6 and zinc. Make sure your diet is nutrient rich and, to be on the safe side, take a multivitamin and mineral supplement every day. It can also help to supplement your diet with 300–500 mg of magnesium each day.

7 Reduce your intake of CASSSA

CASSSA stands for caffeine, alcohol, salt, sugar, saturated fat and additives.

Caffeine in excess appears to worsen PMS, and because it is a diuretic it depletes valuable nutrients.

Alcohol also depletes nutrients and can upset your blood sugar levels and interfere with the liver's ability to detoxify your system.

Salt can contribute to bloating, breast tenderness and high blood pressure.

Sugar has no nutritional value and is a major cause of blood sugar imbalance.

Saturated fat can increase oestrogen levels and lead to weight gain, which is clearly bad news.

Additives, preservatives and chemicals in food all contribute to hormonal imbalance. Always try to eat food in its most natural state and without these added chemicals.

8 Lose excess weight

Several scientists have discovered that the more overweight you are, the more likely you are to suffer from PMS. So if you have got weight to lose, eat more nutritious foods, ditch the high-fat and high-sugar foods, and step up your exercise routine.

9 Chill out

Stress is also implicated in PMS. You are more likely to have worse symptoms of PMS when you are stressed than when you are relaxed. Practise ways of relaxing.

10 Get moving

Exercise can lift your mood as it helps to boost the 'feel-good' chemicals in the brain known as endorphins. Low levels of endorphins have also been implicated in PMS. About half an hour of exercise a day should do the trick. If possible, try to exercise outside in the fresh air to enjoy regular exposure to sunlight.

11 Take chasteberry (agnus castus)

Agnus castus is popular in the treatment of PMS – and no wonder, with research suggesting it can improve symptoms by more than 50 per cent. The recommended dose is 40 drops of tincture to be taken every morning.

12 Focus on the good things in life

Every day focus on the good things in life. Appreciate and be grateful for what surrounds you. Create positive images in your mind. Think your way to a PMS-free life.

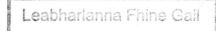

Useful addresses

There are some NHS clinics or support groups for PMS that require a letter of referral from your GP. Some women's health centres have information or support groups as well.

National Association for Premenstrual Syndrome (NAPS)
41 Old Road
East Peckham
Kent TN12 5AP
Helpline: 0870 777 2177
Email: contact@pms.org.uk
Website: www.pms.org.uk

NAPS aims to help women suffering from PMS, and to further research and understanding of PMS. Produces booklets and a quarterly newsletter.

Premenstrual Society (PREMSOC)
PO Box 429
Addlestone
Surrey KT15 1DZ
Tel: 01932 872560 (11 a.m. to 6 p.m., weekdays)

Provides support for PMS self-help groups and individuals; runs courses and publishes a newsletter. Answers general enquiries by phone and post. Send an SAE for information plus publication list.

Women's Nutritional Advisory Service
Natural Health Advisory Service
PO Box 268
Lewes
East Sussex BN7 1QN
Tel: 01273 487366
Fax: 01273 487576
Email: enquiries@naturalhealthas.com
Website: www.naturalhealthas.com

Nutritional treatment for PMS. For a fee, your symptoms, diet, medical history and lifestyle will be analysed and a dietary treatment plan devised. Access to counsellors by phone.

Complementary practitioners

For a list of registered practitioners, send a large SAE to the organizations listed below:

British Acupuncture Council
63 Jeddo Road
London W12 9HQ
Tel: 020 8735 0400
Email: info@acupuncture.co.uk
Website: www.acupuncture.co.uk

British Association for Counselling and Psychotherapy (BACP)
35–37 Albert Street
Rugby
Warwickshire CV21 2SG
Tel: 0870 443 5252
Email: bacp@bacp.co.uk
Website: www.bacp.co.uk

British Association for Nutritional Therapy
27 Old Gloucester Street
London W1N 3XX
Tel: 0870 606 1284
Email: theadministrator@bant.org.uk
Website: www.bant.org.uk

British Complementary Medicine Association (BCMA)
PO Box 5122
Bournemouth BH8 0WG
Tel: 0845 345 5977
Email: info@bcma.co.uk
Website: www.bcma.co.uk

British Wheel of Yoga
25 Jermyn Street
Sleaford
Lincs NG34 7RU
Tel: 01529 306851
Email: office@bwy.org.uk
Website: www.bwy.org.uk

General Council for Massage Therapy
Whiteway House
Blundells Lane
Rainhill
Prescot
Merseyside L35 6NB
Tel: 0870 850 4452
Email: gcmt@btconnect.com
Website: www.gcmt.org.uk

The International Federation of Professional Aromatherapists
82 Ashby Road
Hinckley
Leicestershire LE10 1SN
Tel: 01455 637987
Email: admin@ifparoma.org
Website: www.ifparoma.org

National Institute of Medical Herbalists (NIMH)
Elm House
54 Mary Arches Street
Exeter EX4 3BA
Tel: 01392 426022
Email: nimh@ukexeter.freeserve.co.uk
Website: www.nimh.org.uk

The Register of Chinese Herbal Medicine
Office 5
1 Exeter Street
Norwich
Norfolk NR2 4QB
Tel: 01603 623994

Email: herbmed@rchm.co.uk
Website: www.rchm.co.uk

Transcendental Meditation (Independent) UK
(North) Chris Greathead
Tel: 0191 213 2179
Email: chris@tm-meditation.co.uk
(South) Colin Beckley
Tel: 01843 84010
Email: colin@tm-meditation.co.uk

Telephone for free information pack.

The Women's Clinic
Royal London Homeopathic Hospital
60 Great Ormond Street
London WC1N 3HR
Tel: 0845 155 5000
Website: rlhh.org.uk

Other useful websites

www.womenshealth.com
www.obgyn.upenn.edu/pms/pms.html
www.nlm.nih.gov/medlineplus/menstruationandpremenstrual
    syndrome.html
www.coolpress.com (his and hers PMS calendar)

Further reading

Dalton, Katharina, *PMS: The Essential Guide to Treatment Options.* Thorsons, London, 1994.

Evennett, Karen, *The PMS Diet Book.* Sheldon Press, London, 1997.

Evennett, Karen, *Coping Successfully with PMS.* Sheldon Press, London, 2000.

Glenville, Marilyn, *Natural Solutions to PMS.* Piatkus, London, 2002.

Harris, Colette, and Cheung, Theresa, *You Can Beat PMS: The 12 Week Plan to Banish Symptoms.* Thorsons, London, 2004.

Holford, Patrick, and Neil, Kate, *Balance Hormones Naturally.* Piatkus, London, 1998.

Stewart, Maryon, *No More PMS.* Vermilion, London, 1997.

Notes

1 E. Accorrt et al. (2006) 'Frontal EEG asymmetry and premenstrual dysphoric symptomatology', *Journal of Abnormal Psychology*, February; 115(1): 179–84.
2 A. W. Clare et al. (1985) 'Premenstrual syndrome: single or multiple causes?', *Canadian Journal of Psychiatry*, November; 30(7): 474–82.
3 A. Bendich et al. (2000) 'The potential for dietary supplements to reduce premenstrual syndrome (PMS) symptoms', *Journal of American College of Nutrition*, February; 19(1): 3–12.
4 A. Perk et al. (2004) 'Risk factors for premenstrual dysphoric disorder in a community sample of young women: the role of traumatic events and posttraumatic stress disorder', *Journal of Clinical Psychiatry*, October; 65(10): 1314–22.
5 P. D. Parker et al. (1994) 'Premenstrual syndrome', *American Family Physician*, 1 November; 50(6): 1309–17, 1323–4.
6 'New treatment approaches for premenstrual disorders' (2005) *American Journal of Managed Care*, December; 11(16 Suppl): S480–91.
7 A. Rapkin et al. (2005) 'New treatment approaches for premenstrual disorders', *American Journal of Managed Care*, December; 11(16 Suppl): S480–91; B. Gianetto et al. (2004) 'Soy, fat and other dietary factors in relation to premenstrual symptoms in Japanese women', *British Journal of Obstetrics and Gynaecology*, June; 111(6): 594–9; Elizabeth Bertone-Johnson et al. (2005) 'Calcium and vitamin D intake and risk of incident premenstrual syndrome', *Archives of Internal Medicine*, 13 June; 165(11): 1246–52.
8 A. Ross et al. (1990) 'Caffeine-containing beverages, total fluid consumption, and premenstrual syndrome', *American Journal of Public Health*, September; 80(9): 1106–10.
9 K. Wyatt et al. (1999) 'Efficacy of vitamin B-6 in the treatment of premenstrual syndrome: systematic review', *British Medical Journal*, 22 May; 318(7195): 1375–81.
10 R. London et al. (1983) 'Evaluation and treatment of breast symptoms in patients with the premenstrual syndrome', *Journal*

NOTES

of Reproductive Medicine, August; 28(8): 503–8.

11 Elizabeth Bertone-Johnson et al. (2005) 'Calcium and vitamin D intake and risk of incident premenstrual syndrome', *Archives of Internal Medicine*, 13 June; 165(11): 1246–52.

12 S. Johnson et al. (2001) 'The multifaceted and widespread pathology of magnesium deficiency', *Medical Hypotheses*, February; 56(2): 163–70.

13 W. Johnson et al. (1995) 'Macronutrient intake, eating habits, and exercise as moderators of menstrual distress in healthy women', *Psychosomatic Medicine*, July–August; 57(4): 324–30; J. C. Prior et al. (1986) 'Conditioning exercise decreases premenstrual symptoms. A prospective controlled three month trial', *European Journal of Applied Physiology and Occupational Physiology*; 55(4): 349–55.

14 P. Stran et al. (2002) 'Menstrual cycle, beta-endorphins, and pain sensitivity in premenstrual dysphoric disorder', *Health Psychology*, July; 21(4): 358–67.

15 'The beneficial effect of yoga in diabetes' (2005) *Nepal Medical College Journal*, December; 7(2): 145–7.

16 B. Tesch et al. (2003) 'Herbs commonly used by women: an evidence-based review', *American Journal of Obstetrics and Gynecology*, May; 188(5 Suppl): S44–55; 'Herbal treatment for PMS' (2001) *Harvard Women's Health Watch*, May; 8(9): 7.

17 R. Schellenberg (2001) 'Treatment for the pre-menstrual syndrome with agnus fruit extract: perspective, randomized, placebo controlled trials', *British Medical Journal*, 322: 134–7.

18 S. J. Sheu et al. (1987) 'Analysis and processing of Chinese herbal drugs IV: The Study of Angelicae radix', *Planta Medica*, 53: 377–8; M. Qi-bing et al. (1991) 'Advance in the pharmacological studies of radix Angelic sinensis', *Chinese Medical Journal*, 104: 776–81.

19 I. J. McFayden et al. (1992) 'Cyclical breast pain – some observations and the difficulties in treatment', *British Journal of Clinical Practice*, 46: 161–4.

20 S. Masho (2005) 'Obesity as a risk factor for premenstrual syndrome', *Journal of Psychosomatic Obstetrics and Gynaecology*, March; 26(1): 33–9.

21 A. Perk et al. (2004) 'Risk factors for premenstrual dysphoric disorder in a community sample of young women: the role of traumatic events and posttraumatic stress disorder', *Journal of*

Psychiatry, October; 65(10): 1314–22.
22 K. Shin et al. (2000) 'Menstrual changes in sleep, rectal temperature and melatonin rhythms in a subject with premenstrual syndrome', *Neuroscience Letters*, 10 March; 281(2–3): 159–62.
23 A. Girman et al. (2003) 'An integrative medicine approach to premenstrual syndrome', *American Journal of Obstetrics and Gynaecology*, May; 188(5 Suppl): S56–65.
24 A. Jones et al. (2003) 'Homeopathic treatment for premenstrual symptoms', *Journal of Family Planning and Reproductive Health Care*, January; 29(1): 25–8.
25 K. Shin et al. (2000) 'Menstrual changes in sleep, rectal temperature and melatonin rhythms in a subject with premenstrual syndrome' (2000) *Neuroscience Letters*, 10 March; 281(2–3): 159–62.
26 N. Chen (1996) 'Individual differences in answering the four questions for happiness', PhD dissertation, University of Georgia, Athens, Georgia.
27 N. F. Woods et al. (1985) 'Major life events, daily stressors and perimenstrual symptoms', *Nursing Research*, 34: 263–7.
28 K. R. Fontaine et al. (1997) 'Optimism, social support and premenstrual dysphoria', *Journal of Clinical Psychology*, 53: 243–7; G. Morse (1999) 'Positively reframing perceptions of the menstrual cycle among women with premenstrual syndrome', *Journal of Obstetrics, Gynecologic and Neonatal Nursing*, 28: 165–74.
29 B. Snider and D. Dieteman (1974) 'Pyridoxine therapy for premenstrual acne flare up', *Archives of Dermatology*, 110: 130–1.
30 O. Janiger et al. (1972) 'Cross cultural study of PMS symptoms', *Psychosomatics*, 13: 226–35.
31 N. L. Petrakis et al. (1981) 'Cytological abnormalities in nipple aspirates of breast fluid from women with severe constipation', *Lancet*, 2(8257): 1203–4.
32 R. London et al. (1982) 'Mammary dysplasia: Endocrine parameters and tocopherol therapy', *Nutrition Research*, 7: 243.
33 I. J. McFayden et al. (1992) 'Cyclical breast pain – some observations and the difficulties in treatment', *British Journal of Clinical Practice*, 46: 161–4.
34 A. Tamborini et al. (1993) 'Value of standardized ginkgo biloba extract (EGb 761) in the management of congestive symptoms of

premenstrual syndrome', *Revue Francaise de gynecologie et d'obstetrique*, July–September, 88(7–9): 447–57.

35 K. Dalton (1960) 'Menstruation and accidents', *British Medical Journal*, 2: 1425–6.

36 A. Tamborini et al. (1993) 'Value of standardized ginkgo biloba extract (EGb 761) in the management of congestive symptoms of premenstrual syndrome', *Revue Francaise de gynecologie*, July –September, 88(7–9): 447–57.

37 F. Faccinetti et al. (1991) 'Magnesium prophylaxis of menstrual migraine: effects of intracellular magnesium', *Headache*, 31: 298–304.

38 C. J. Glucek et al. (1986) 'Amelioration of severe migraine with Omega 3 fatty acids: A double blind, placebo controlled clinical trial', *American Journal of Clinical Nutrition*, 43: 710.

39 E. S. Johnson et al. (1985) 'Efficacy of feverfew as prophylactic treatment of migraine', *British Medical Journal*, 291: 569–73.

Index